Sara Brittingham

Downregulation of endogenous TRAIL and its effect on cancer cells

AF061807

Sara Brittingham

Downregulation of endogenous TRAIL and its effect on cancer cells

An experimental study

Südwestdeutscher Verlag für Hochschulschriften

Impressum/Imprint (nur für Deutschland/only for Germany)
Bibliografische Information der Deutschen Nationalbibliothek: Die Deutsche Nationalbibliothek verzeichnet diese Publikation in der Deutschen Nationalbibliografie; detaillierte bibliografische Daten sind im Internet über http://dnb.d-nb.de abrufbar.
Alle in diesem Buch genannten Marken und Produktnamen unterliegen warenzeichen-, marken- oder patentrechtlichem Schutz bzw. sind Warenzeichen oder eingetragene Warenzeichen der jeweiligen Inhaber. Die Wiedergabe von Marken, Produktnamen, Gebrauchsnamen, Handelsnamen, Warenbezeichnungen u.s.w. in diesem Werk berechtigt auch ohne besondere Kennzeichnung nicht zu der Annahme, dass solche Namen im Sinne der Warenzeichen- und Markenschutzgesetzgebung als frei zu betrachten wären und daher von jedermann benutzt werden dürften.

Verlag: Südwestdeutscher Verlag für Hochschulschriften GmbH & Co. KG
Heinrich-Böcking-Str. 6-8, 66121 Saarbrücken, Deutschland
Telefon +49 681 37 20 271-1, Telefax +49 681 37 20 271-0
Email: info@svh-verlag.de

Approved by: München, LMU, Dissertation, 2011

Herstellung in Deutschland:
Schaltungsdienst Lange o.H.G., Berlin
Books on Demand GmbH, Norderstedt
Reha GmbH, Saarbrücken
Amazon Distribution GmbH, Leipzig
ISBN: 978-3-8381-3105-4

Imprint (only for USA, GB)
Bibliographic information published by the Deutsche Nationalbibliothek: The Deutsche Nationalbibliothek lists this publication in the Deutsche Nationalbibliografie; detailed bibliographic data are available in the Internet at http://dnb.d-nb.de.
Any brand names and product names mentioned in this book are subject to trademark, brand or patent protection and are trademarks or registered trademarks of their respective holders. The use of brand names, product names, common names, trade names, product descriptions etc. even without a particular marking in this works is in no way to be construed to mean that such names may be regarded as unrestricted in respect of trademark and brand protection legislation and could thus be used by anyone.

Publisher: Südwestdeutscher Verlag für Hochschulschriften GmbH & Co. KG
Heinrich-Böcking-Str. 6-8, 66121 Saarbrücken, Germany
Phone +49 681 37 20 271-1, Fax +49 681 37 20 271-0
Email: info@svh-verlag.de

Printed in the U.S.A.
Printed in the U.K. by (see last page)
ISBN: 978-3-8381-3105-4

Copyright © 2012 by the author and Südwestdeutscher Verlag für Hochschulschriften GmbH & Co. KG and licensors
All rights reserved. Saarbrücken 2012

1 INDEX

1 INDEX	1
2 ABBREVIATIONS	4
3 INTRODUCTION	5
3.1 BACKGROUND	5
3.2 MULTIPLE BIOLOGICAL FUNCTIONS OF TRAIL	6
3.3 EXPRESSION OF TUMOR NECROSIS FACTOR-RELATED APOPTOSIS-INDUCING LIGAND (TRAIL)	7
3.4 TRAIL AND ITS RECEPTORS	7
3.5 APOPTOSIS AND THE PRO-APOPTOTIC EFFECT OF TRAIL	8
3.6 TRAIL AS AN ANTI-CANCER DRUG	10
3.7 NON-APOPTOTIC EFFECT OF TRAIL	11
3.8 THE PRO-PROLIFERATIVE EFFECT OF TRAIL	12
3.9 AIM OF PRESENT WORK	13
4 MATERIAL	14
4.1 CELL LINES	14
4.2 OLIGONUCLEOTIDES	15
4.3 ANTIBODIES OF WESTERN BLOT ANALYSIS	16
4.4 KITS	16
4.5 SOFTWARE	16
4.6 LABORATORY EQUIPEMENT	17
4.7 MATERIALS OF CELL CULTURE	18
4.8 CHEMICALS	19
4.9 SOLUTIONS/ BUFFERS	20
5 METHODS	21
5.1 CELL CULTURE	21
5.2 IN-VITRO ASSAYS	21
5.2.1 Stimulation with TRAIL	21

Index

5.2.2	Transient transfection	22
5.2.3	Caspase inhibition	23

5.3 CELL GROWTH ANALYSIS USING CELLSCREEN ... 23
5.4 CELL DEATH ANALYSIS USING FLUORESCENCE ACTIVATED CELL SORTING (FACS) ... 24
5.5 ANALYSIS OF TRANSFECTION EFFICIENCY USING FLUORESCENCE ACTIVATED CELL SORTING (FACS) ... 25
5.6 STATISTICAL ANALYSIS ... 25
5.7 RNA/DNA STUDIES ... 26

- 5.7.1 RNA Isolation and quantification ... 26
- 5.7.2 Reverse Transcriptase Reaction ... 26
- 5.7.3 Quantitative Real-Time Polymerase Chain Reaction (qRT-PCR) ... 27
- 5.7.4 Analysis of qRT-PCR (crossing point and melting curve analysis) ... 28

5.8 PROTEIN STUDIES ... 30

- 5.8.1 Cell lysis ... 30
- 5.8.2 SDS-Polyacrylamid Gel Electrophoresis (PAGE) ... 31
- 5.8.3 Immunoblotting and Immunodetection ... 32

6 RESULTS ... 33

6.1 TRAIL MEDIATED PROLIFERATION ... 33
6.2 DOWNREGULATION OF ENDOGENOUS TRAIL: OPTIMIZATION ... 35

- 6.2.1 Screening human cell lines for endogenous TRAIL expression ... 35
- 6.2.2 Evaluation of siRNA delivery ... 37
- 6.2.3 Evaluation of siRNA efficiency ... 39
  - 6.2.3.1 Efficiency on RNA level ... 39
  - 6.2.3.2 Efficiency on Protein Level ... 41

6.3 DOWNREGULATION OF ENDOGENOUS TRAIL: SCREENING FOR EFFECTS ON CELL GROWTH 42
6.4 KELLY CELLS AND THE EFFECTS OF DOWNREGULATION OF ENDOGENOUS TRAIL ... 48

- 6.4.1 Reduction of cell growth ... 48
- 6.4.2 Cell growth reduction is a result of cell death induction ... 51
- 6.4.3 Soluble TRAIL rescues cell death induced by the downregulation of endogenous TRAIL ... 54

Index

    6.4.4   Cell death is mediated by caspases 56

7   DISCUSSION 59

    7.1   SUBSTANTIAL EFFECT OF THE DOWN REGULATION OF TRAIL ON CELL VIABILITY 59

    7.2   CELL-TYPE SPECIFICITY OF THE FUNCTION OF ENDOGENOUS TRAIL 60

    7.3   ROLE OF ENDOGENOUS TRAIL FOR CANCER CELLS 61

    7.4   PRO-SURVIVAL FUNCTION OF SEVERAL MEMBERS OF THE TNF-FAMILY 62

    7.5   MECHANISMS OF THE PRO-SURVIVAL FUNCTION OF TNF-FAMILY MEMBERS 63

    7.6   FUTURE PERSPECTIVE 64

    7.7   POTENTIAL RELEVANCE AS A NOVEL APPROACH OF CANCER THERAPY 64

8   SUMMARY 65

9   ZUSAMMENFASSUNG 66

10 REFERENCES 67

11 ACKNOWLEDGEMENT 75

12 PUBLICATION 76

Index

2 Abbreviations

A	Adenosine
Ab	Antibody
BSA	Bovine Serum Albumin
C	Cytosine
cDNA	Complementary DNA
Conc	Concentration
DMEM	Dubeco's minimum essential medium
DMSO	Dimethylsulfoxid
DNA	Desoxyribonucleotide triphosphate
FAM	Carboxyfluorescein
FCS	Fetal Calf Serum
FSC	Forward Scatter
G	Guanin
GAPDH	Glycerinaldehyd-3-phosphat-dehydrogenase
HPRT	Hypoxanthin-Guanin-Phosphoribosyltransferase
kDa	Kilo Dalton
mRNA	Messenger ribonuclein acid
SSC	Sideward Scatter
siRNA	Small interfering RNA
T	Thymidine
Tab	Table
TNF/TNFR	Tumor necrosis factor/ Tumor necrosis factor receptor
TRAIL	Tumor necrosis factor related apoptosis inducing ligand
TRAIL-R	TRAIL-Receptor
U	Uracil

3 Introduction

3.1 Background

Cancer is one of the leading causes of death (Ferlay et al., 2010). Cancer therapy attracts considerable research attention and has made great advances in past decades. The aim of cancer therapy is to effectively reduce the amount of malignant tumor cells while sparing healthy cells. To reach this goal cancer therapy has become an interdisciplinary field. Today it incorporates the field of Surgery, Radiotherapy, Chemotherapy and Immunotherapy (Neubauer et al., 2002). In most advanced cancers chemotherapy plays an integral role (Papac, 2001). Cytotoxic drugs applied in chemotherapy exert high toxicity on tumor cells. In general most healthy cells are not spared from cell death. Adverse effects of chemotherapy are linked to the toxicity of cytotoxic drugs on healthy cells. Multiple adverse effects have been described, ranging from hair loss, diarrhea to more life threatening myelosuppression and organ failure. These adverse effects limit the effectiveness of cancer therapy in advanced stage cancer disease. The search for novel strategies of selective cancer therapy as well as the search for novel anti-cancer drugs with minimal adverse effects is ongoing. In the past, several drugs have been proposed as potential new anti-cancer drugs (Caponigro et al., 2005). Among the newly identified anti-cancer drugs Tumor necrosis factor related apoptosis-inducing ligand (TRAIL) was found to selectively trigger apoptosis in cancer cells (Walczak et al., 1999), while sparing healthy cells (Ashkenazi et al., 1999). But in depth research in our laboratory detected an unexpected adverse effect of TRAIL. TRAIL improved survival and accelerated cell growth on a subset of TRAIL resistant cancers (Ehrhardt et al., 2003; Baader et al., 2005). The pro-proliferative effect of TRAIL opposed the initially described function of TRAIL and represented a threat for a successful cancer therapy.

Introduction

3.2 Multiple biological functions of TRAIL

Independently isolated by Pitti and Wiley (Wiley et al., 1995; Pitti et al., 1996) Tumor necrosis factor related apoptosis-inducing ligand (TRAIL), also called Apo2 ligand, was identified as a member of the tumor necrosis factor superfamily (TNFSF), a group of proteins involved in the regulation of the immune system (Gruss and Dower, 1995).

Since its discovery multiple biological functions of TRAIL have been proposed (Levina et al., 2008). The significance of TRAIL for innate immunity has been emphasized, showing that the up regulation of TRAIL in lung tissue accelerated clearance of viral infections in mice, e.g. with influenza virus, (Ishikawa et al., 2005). In Natural Killer cells TRAIL cell activation was associated with an up regulation of surface bound TRAIL (Smyth et al., 2001; Street et al., 2001). Other reports provided evidence for the involvement of TRAIL in autoimmune disease. TRAIL-deficient mice showed defective thymocyte development and increased sensitivity to autoimmune disease (Lamhamedi-Cherradi et al., 2003). In-vivo studies provided data that recombinant TRAIL induced pathognomonic features of asthma and promoted eosinophilic survival in mice, underlining a role of TRAIL in the field of allergology (Robertson et al., 2002; Weckmann et al., 2007).

In addition TRAIL was found to have a considerable role for tumor biology. Both tumor formation and tumor metastasis were found to be controlled by TRAIL. Studies showed the potential of TRAIL as a pro-apoptotic factor, suppressing tumor cell growth (Shi et al., 2005) and tumor metastasis in-vivo (Grosse-Wilde and Kemp, 2008). Yet a key role as a suppressor of tumor genesis could not be successfully established. In-vivo studies on TRAIL-deficient mice failed to show spontaneous formation of tumors (Sedger et al., 2002).

Introduction

3.3 Expression of Tumor necrosis factor-related apoptosis-inducing ligand (TRAIL)

TRAIL was initially found to be expressed on activated cells of the immune system, among them dendritic cells (Fanger *et al.*, 1999), NK cells, monocytes and resting T-cells (Kayagaki *et al.*, 1999). A tissue-wide screen further identified a variety of transformed and non-transformed organs expressing TRAIL (Wiley *et al.*, 1995; Spierings *et al.*, 2004). The expression of TRAIL was described as a prognostic factor for several solid cancers, including end stage colon cancer (Van Geelen *et al.*, 2006), renal cell cancer (Macher-Goeppinger *et al.*, 2009), end stage lung cancer (Spierings *et al.*, 2003), melanoma (Bron *et al.*, 2004) and gynecological cancers such as ovarian cancer (Lancaster *et al.*, 2003), breast cancer (Van *et al.*, 2006) and cervical cancer (Maduro *et al.*, 2009). Furthermore endogenous TRAIL expression was shown to be regulated by different factors. For instance, INF-gamma, a cytokine with an important role for innate and adaptive immunity, up-regulates the expression of TRAIL on inflammatory cells (Smyth *et al.*, 2001; Abadie and Wietzerbin, 2003). Immunostimulants, such as viral RNA or synthetic double stranded analogs, for instance Poly (I:C), and Lipopolysaccharin (LPS), a bacterial endotoxin, have also been shown to have an up-regulatory effect on TRAIL expression (Halaas *et al.*, 2004; Harada *et al.*, 2007; Cho *et al.*, 2010).

3.4 TRAIL and its receptors

TRAIL is expressed as a type 2 transmembrane protein, with an intracellular amino-terminal region, a transmembrane domain and an extracellular carboxy terminal region (Wiley *et al.*, 1995). TRAIL remains surface-bound or, alternatively, its extracellular domain is proteolytically cleaved from the cell surface or is released in association with micro vesicles to produce soluble TRAIL (Wiley *et al.*, 1995; Martinez-Lorenzo *et al.*, 1999). Both surface bound TRAIL and soluble TRAIL interact in humans with five receptors, among them death receptor 4, 5 (DR-4 / DR-5), decoy receptor 1, 2 (DcR-1 / DcR-2) and osteoprotegerin (OPG) (Mongkolsapaya *et al.*, 1999). DR-4 (TRAIL-R1) and DR-5 (TRAIL-R2) belong to the TNF receptor family and hold a death domain. Both death receptors induce cell death upon binding with TRAIL (Pan *et al.*, 1997; Sheridan *et al.*, 1997). TRAIL also binds to DcR-1 / DcR-2, which are closely related to DR4 and 5, but do not induce cell death due to structural differences within the receptor. DcR-1 lacks a cytosolic region which is necessary to transfer

Introduction

the death signal (Sheridan *et al.*, 1997). DcR2 has a truncated non-functioning cytosolic death domain which prevents further death signaling (Marsters *et al.*, 1997). In addition to the death receptors TRAIL binds with low affinity to the soluble TNF receptor family member osteoprotegerin (OPG). The significance of its binding remains poorly understood up-to-date (Kimberley and Screaton, 2004).

3.5 Apoptosis and the pro-apoptotic effect of TRAIL

Apoptosis is a cell´s intrinsic death program which demarcates itself from other forms of cell death, for instance necrosis, as a programmed and deliberate mode of cell dying. Apoptosis is characterized by typical morphological changes, such as cell shrinkage, nuclear defragmentation and membrane blebbing (Hengartner, 2000). Important effector molecules of apoptosis are proteolytically active enzymes, which are termed caspases (Degterev *et al.*, 2003). Chemotherapeutic agents, among them TRAIL, contribute to the activation of caspases by initiating the extrinsic or intrinsic pathway of apoptosis (Fulda and Debatin, 2004).

A well known extrinsic stimulus for the induction of apoptosis is the interaction of TRAIL with its cellular death receptors, DR-4 (TRAIL Receptors 1) and DR-5 (TRAIL Receptors 2). The interaction of TRAIL with its death receptors initiates an intracellular molecular cascade which concludes with apoptotic cell death. The binding of TRAIL with its receptor induces the clustering of the receptor´s death domain and the recruitment of the adapter molecule Fas-associated death domain (FADD) (Walczek and Krammer, 2000). FADD in turns recruits caspase 8, which serves as the apoptosis initiator and forms the so called death- inducing signaling complex (DISC) (Kischkel *et al.*, 1995; Sprick *et al.*, 2000). Initiator caspases activate a cascade of downstream caspases, termed the effector caspases, leading eventually to features of apoptosis, such as the degradation of cytoplasmatic proteins and the fragmentation of nuclear DNA (Ashkenazi, 2002). Figure 1 illustrates the intracellular cascade of the extrinsic pathway of apoptosis.

Introduction

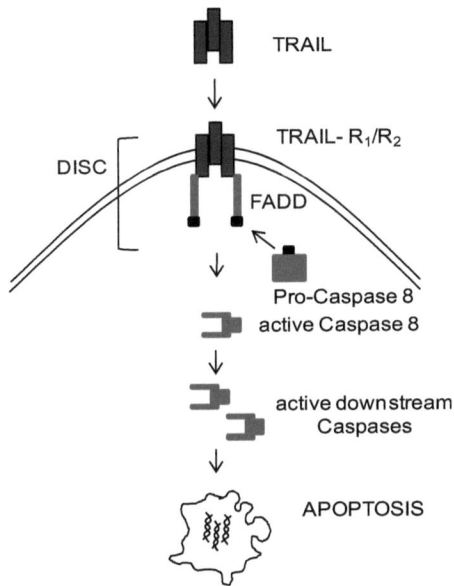

Figure 1. TRAIL activates the extrinsic pathway of apoptosis by binding TRAIL receptor R_1/R_2. (Modeled after "TRAIL signaling: Decisions between life and death", (Falschlehner et al., 2007)).

Next to extrinsic stimuli which activate the extrinsic pathway of apoptosis intrinsic stimuli can function as initiators of apoptosis. Apoptosis induction through the intrinsic pathway is mediated partly by mitochondrial activation. Various chemotherapeutic agents induce mitochondrial damage by disrupting the mitochondrial membrane and by increasing membrane permeability (Decaudin et al., 1998; Green and Kroemer, 2004). A consequence of increased membrane permeability is the release of proteins which normally occupy the space between mitochondrial inner and outer membrane. These proteins, among them cytochrome c, once in the cytoplasm, activate the aforementioned cascade of caspases or carry out a caspase independent death program (Saelens et al., 2004).

Introduction

3.6 TRAIL as an anti-cancer drug

Apoptosis plays a major role in regulating tumor formation (Fulda and Debatin, 2006). TRAIL's role as an anti cancer drug has been emphasized in in-vitro studies which showed that TRAIL induces cell death in cancer cells (Walczak et al., 1999), while sparing normal cells (Ashkenazi et al., 1999). A variety of cancers, both liquid and solid cancers, have been described sensitive to TRAIL therapy in in-vivo experiments. The systemic administration of TRAIL showed decreased tumor growth in murine xenograft models of colon carcinoma (Kelley et al., 2001), models of breast carcinoma (Walczak et al., 1999), malignant glioma (Roth et al., 1999) and thyroid cancer (Ahmad and Shi, 2000). Even tumors with high resistance to conventional cytostatics drugs, particularly multiple myeloma, were effectively treated with TRAIL therapy (Mitsiades et al., 2001). The tumoricidal effect of TRAIL is effectively increased when applied in combination with other cytostatic drugs. In human glioma and acute leukemia combination therapy with TRAIL markedly increased cell death, which was attributed to an upregulation of DR5 in tumor cells (Nagane et al., 2000; Wen et al., 2000). Increased efficiency of chemotherapy was also seen in human breast carcinoma and hepatocellular carcinoma, conferring TRAIL the role of a sensitizing agent (Keane et al., 1999; Ganten et al., 2004). The sensitizing effect of TRAIL was further observed in conjunction with radiation therapy in lymphoma cells (Belka et al., 2001). Next to its apoptosis inducing effect on cancer cells, TRAIL's ability to spare healthy cells emphasizes its potential as an anti-cancer drug. Normal fibroblasts, epithelial cells, astrocytes and smooth muscle cells were not affected by the cytotoxicity of TRAIL (Ashkenazi et al., 1999). Reports proposed a toxic effect of TRAIL on neurons in the presence of ischemia and hepatocytes (Martin-Villalba et al., 1999; Jo et al., 2000), but subsequent studies contained the risk reporting that cytotoxicity of hepatocytes was attributed to the high dose and to the derivative of TRAIL applied in the study (LeBlanc and Ashkenazi, 2003).

3.7 Non-apoptotic effect of TRAIL

TRAIL´s rising potential as an anti-cancer drug was damped by an increasing occurrence of resistance to TRAIL therapy. A significant number of cancer cell lines and tumors showed resistance to TRAIL induced apoptosis (Kim *et al.*, 2000) or became resistant to the apoptosis inducing effect of TRAIL through prolonged or repeated exposure to TRAIL (acquired resistance). For example, human invasive neuroblastoma cell lines (Hopkins-Donaldson *et al.*, 2000) and renal cell cancer (Oya *et al.*, 2001) did not respond to apoptosis when treated with TRAIL, while for instance breast cancer cells became resistant to TRAIL when incubated with repeated sub toxic doses of TRAIL (Yoshida *et al.*, 2009). A screening of human urothelial carcinoma cell lines showed that 2 out of 6 cell lines were resistant or refractory to the apoptosis inducing effect of TRAIL. Further studies were conducted in our research lab on leukemic cells and solid tumor cell lines. A screening of 53 leukemic samples, which were obtained from children with newly diagnosed acute leukemia, showed that 73% of patients were resistant to TRAIL induced apoptosis. Lower numbers were obtained from the screening of solid tumor cell lines subjected to TRAIL treatment. Among 18 cell lines tested, 56% showed sensitivity, 44% showed resistance to TRAIL induced apoptosis. The study went on to examine TRAIL resistance in cancer cell lines in more detail. Four of 18 cancer cell lines revealed an unexpected increase in cell growth and survival upon TRAIL treatment (Baader *et al.*, 2005).

Introduction

3.8 The pro-proliferative effect of TRAIL

Up-to-date TRAIL mediated proliferation has been identified on a group of TRAIL resistant cancer cells including human leukemia cells (Ehrhardt et al., 2003), human neuroblastoma cells (Baader et al., 2005), pancreatic cancer (Trauzold et al., 2006), human small cell lung carcinoma (Belyanskaya et al., 2008) and human glioma cells (Vilimanovich and Bumbasirevic et al., 2008). In-vitro studies further extended the observed pro-proliferative, pro-survival effect of soluble TRAIL to non-cancerous cells such as t-lymphocytes (Chou et al., 2001), vascular endothelial cells (Secchiero et al., 2004) and synovial fibroblasts (Morel et al., 2005). Furthermore, clinical studies described an association of increased endogenous TRAIL expression and decreased disease-specific survival in renal cell carcinoma and cholangiocarcinoma (Macher-Goeppinger et al., 2009; Ishimura et al., 2006), proposing a tumor promoting role of endogenous TRAIL. Throughout the tumor entities different molecular mechanisms were found to be involved in TRAIL mediated proliferation. TRAIL resistant cancer cells which showed TRAIL mediated proliferation formed a heterogeneous cancer group, in which soluble TRAIL exerted a pleiotropic effect. For instance in small cell lung carcinoma cells TRAIL induced proliferation was found to be a result of the activation of ERK, a growth promoting intracellular kinase (Belyanskaya et al., 2008). In human vascular endothelial cells growth induced by soluble TRAIL was attributed to the activation of Akt, a growth regulating serine/threonine kinase (Secchiero et al., 2003). Furthermore the transcription factor NF-κB, an activator of pro-inflammatory and pro-proliferative genes and key regulator of cell growth (Karin et al., 2002) was described to be involved in TRAIL induced proliferation in lymphoid cells and cells of cholangiocarcinoma (Malhi and Gores, 2006). Studies on lymphoid cells showed the activation of NF-κB upon binding of TRAIL to its receptors (Lin et al., 2000; Ehrhardt et al., 2003; Zauli et al., 2005). The concomitant inhibition of NF-κB during TRAIL treatment eliminated TRAIL induced proliferation (Jeremias and Debatin, 1998). In cholangiocarcinoma cells the importance of the activation of NF-κB for TRAIL induced cell migration and tumor invasion was observed (Ishimura et al., 2006).

Introduction

3.9 Aim of present work

The present work is based on published data showing that TRAIL can induce survival and proliferation in human neuroblastoma, small cell lung cancer and cholangiocarcinoma cells (Ehrhardt *et al.*, 2003, Baader *et al.*, 2005; Belyanskaya *et al.*, 2008). The growth promoting effect of soluble TRAIL implicates a possible role of endogenous TRAIL as an endogenous growth factor in cancers resistant to TRAIL-induced apoptosis.

Therefore, the present work had the aim to study the role of endogenous TRAIL for spontaneous cell growth and survival in cancer cells resistant to TRAIL-induced apoptosis. Towards this aim, the expression levels of endogenous TRAIL were reduced using RNA interference. In a first step, the transfection method was optimized together with the confirmatory readouts of successful knockdown. In a second step, these techniques were used to knockdown endogenous TRAIL in the neuroblastoma cell line KELLY, a cancer cell line resistant towards TRAIL-induced apoptosis. In addition, two cancer cell lines, sensitive towards TRAIL-induced apoptosis, were subjected to the knockdown of endogenous TRAIL. Functional readouts for growth and apoptosis finally enabled to determine the impact of endogenous TRAIL for each of these cell lines.

Taken together, the presenting work had the aim to evaluate the putative role of endogenous TRAIL as a novel therapeutic target in the therapy of cancers resistant to TRAIL-induced apoptosis.

4 Material

4.1 Cell lines

Adherent cell lines used in this work were of human origin.
Table below describes cell lines applied in this work:

Name of cell line	Cell type and origin	Morphology	P*
KELLY	Neuroblastoma cell line (Fulda *et al.*, 2001)	Adherent	1:3
SHEP	Neuroblastoma cell line (Baader *et al.*, 2005)	Adherent	1:3
HEK 293	Embryonic kidney tissue (EKT) cell line (Shetty *et al.*, 2002)	Adherent	1:10
HEKpCDNA.TRAIL	EKT cell line stabily transfected with pCDA-vector (Hausherr-Bohn, 2009)	Adherent	1:10
Melanoma 1205 Lu	Lung metastasized melanoma cell line (Besch *et al.*, 2009)	Adherent	1:10

P*= dilution ratio after passaging

Material

4.2 Oligonucleotides

Oligonucleotides (siRNAs and primers) used in this work were obtained from MWG-Biotech. Immunostimulant, Poly (I:C), was a kind gift of Dr. Robert Besch. All oligonucleotides were stored at -20° C.

Small interfering RNAs (siRNAs)

Name	Sequence	Modification	Conc.
TRAIL787	5`GGU CUA AAG AUG CAG AAU ATT 3`	None	20 µM
TRAIL127	5`GCA GAU GCA GGA CAA GUA CTT 3`	None	20 µM
TRAILq2	5`AAC ACA AAG AAC GAC AAA CAA 3`	None	20 µM
LAMIN	5`ACU GCA GCA UCA UGA AAU CTT 3`	None	20 µM
LAMINFAM	5`ACU GCA GCA UCA UGA AAU CTT 3`	5`FAM	20 µM
TRAIL787FAM	5`GGU CUA AAG AUG CAG AAU ATT 3`	5`FAM	20 µM

Primers

Name	Direction	Sequence	Type	Conc.
TRAIL	Reverse	5`TCT TGG AGT TTG GAG AAG AC 3`	Target	0.5 µM
TRAIL	Forward	5`GTC AGC TCG TAA GAA AGA TG 3`	Target	0.5 µM
HPRT	Reverse	5`AGG AAA GCA AAG TCT GCA TT 3`	Control	0.5 µM
HPRT	Forward	5`GGT GGA GAT GAT CTC TCA AC 3`	Control	0.5 µM

Immunostimulant

Name	Conc.
Polyinosinic-polycytidylic acid (Poly(I:C))	3 µM (Besch et al., 2009)

Material

4.3 Antibodies of Western blot analysis

Name	Species	Dilution	Origin
Anti-TRAIL	Rabbit	1:200 in 5% milk	Peprotech
Anti-GAPDH	Mouse	1: 20.000 in TBST	Affinity Bioreagents
Anti-Mouse (2. Ab)	Goat	1:20.000 in TBST	Pierce
Anti-Rabbit (2.Ab)	Goat	1:5000 in Rotiblock	Pierce

4.4 Kits

High Capacity cDNA - Reverse Transcription	Applied Biosystems (Foster City, USA)
Light cycler Fast Start DNA - Master Plus SYBR Green	Roche (Mannheim, D)
SV total RNA Isolation System	Promega (Madison, USA)

4.5 Software

Cell Quest Pro	BD Biosciences (USA)
Excell	Microsoft (Redmond, USA)
Light cycler Software 4.05	Roche (Mannheim, D)
PA Adhesion Software	Innovatis (Bielefeld, D)
SigmaStat	Blue Stallion Tech (South Africa)

Material

4.6 Laboratory Equipement

Cell culture CO_2 Incubator	Heraeus (Hanau, D)
CellScreen	Innovatis (Bielefeld, D)
Centrifuge	Eppendorf (Hamburg, D)
Electrophoresis chamber	Biorad (Hamburg, D)
Filmentwicklungsmaschine	
CP 1000	Agfa (Köln, D)
FACS	Becton Dickinson (Heidelberg, D)
Laminar flow	Heraeus (Hanau, D)
Lightcycler	Roche Diagnostics (Mannheim, D)
Light microscope Olympus	Zeiss (Jena, D)
Nanodrop-ND 2000	Thermoscientific (Bonn, D)
Neubauer counting chamber	Labor Optik (Bad Homburg, D)
Nitrocellulose-membrane	Millipore (Bedford, USA)
PCR cycler	Peqlab (Erlangen, D)
PCR workstation	Peqlab (Erlangen, D)
Pipettes	Eppendorf (Hamburg, D)
Trans-Blot SD semi-dry transfer cell	Biorad (Krefeld, D)
Whatman-paper	BioRad (München, D)

Material

4.7 Materials of cell culture

BSA	Sigma (Steinheim, D)
Cell Culture Flask	BD Bioscience (Heidelberg, D)
DMSO	Sigma (Steinheim, D)
DMEM	Gibco, (San Diego, USA)
FCS	Invitrogen (San Diego, USA)
Ficoll-Isoplaque	Amersham (Uppsala, Sweden)
Gentamycin	Biochrom AG (Berlin, D)
Glutamin	Gibco (San Diego, USA)
Lipofectamine 2000	Invitrogen (Carlsbad, USA)
Lipofectamine RNAimax	Invitrogen (Carlsbad, USA)
L-Glutamin	Gibco (San Diego, USA)
Opti-MEM	Gibco (San Diego, USA)
Penicillin/ Streptomycin	Gibco (San Diego, USA)
Q-vad (10mM solution in DMSO)	Calbiochem (Gibstown, USA)
RPMI Medium1640	Gibco (San Diego, USA)
TRAIL	Peprotech (Rocky Hill, USA)
Trypsin-EDTA	PAN^{TM} Biotech (Aidenbach, D)
24-well plates	BD Bioscience (Heidelberg, D)

*Prior to application FCS was heated to 54 degrees for 30 min

Material

4.8 Chemicals

APS	Biomol (Hamburg, D)
Ethanol	Roth (Karlsruhe, D)
Isopropanol	Roth (Karlsruhe, D)
Methanol	Roth (Karlsruhe, D)
Milchpulver	Roth (Karlsruhe, D)
Page Ruler Prestained	Fermentas (Burlington, USA)
Polyacrylamid 30%	Roth (Karlsruhe, D)
Propidium iodide	Sigma (Steinheim, D)
Protein Ladder	New England Biolabs (Ipswich, USA)
Roti-Block	Roth (Karlsruhe, D)
Rotiphorese Gel 30	Roth (Karlsruhe, D)
SDS	ICN Biomedicals (Meckenheim, D)
TEMED	Roth (Karlsruhe, D)
TRIS	Roth (Karlsruhe, D)
Tween 20	Sigma (Steinheim, D)

Material

4.9 Solutions/ buffers

Buffer A:	36.3 g TRIS (3M), 48 mL 1M HCl, with aqua dest. ad 100 mL, pH = 8.9
Buffer B:	5.7 g TRIS (0.47M), 25.6 mL 1M phosphoric acid, with aqua dest. ad 100 mL, pH = 6.7
Cytosolic lysis-buffer	62.5 mM TRIS-HCl (pH = 6.8), 2% SDS, 10% (1x SDS sample buffer, Glycerin, 0.01% Bromphenolblue cell signaling)
5x loading buffer	12.5 mL 1M TRIS (pH 6,8), 25 mL SDS 20%, 25 mL Glycerol 100%, 12.5 mL aqua ad injectionem
Nicoletti buffer	0.1% Triton-x-100, 0.1% Na-Citrate ad 1 liter water
10x PBS	29.2 g Na_2HPO_4 $2H_2O$, 4 g KH_2PO_4, 160 g NaCl, 4 g KCl, H_2O dd. ad 2 L
5x running buffer	37.75 g Tris Base, 235 g Glycin, 125 ml SDS (10%)
10x TBS	48.4 g TRIS, 60 g NaCl, aqua dest. ad 2 L, pH = 6.8
Transfer buffer	15 g Tris, 71 g Glycin, 790 g Methanol, dest. aqua ad.5L

5 Methods

5.1 Cell culture

All cell culture steps were performed under sterile condition within a laminar flow work station. Cell lines applied in this work (see chapter 4.1) were maintained in RPMI 1620 medium supplemented with 10% FCS and 2 mmol/L L-Glutamine in medium sized culture flasks (75cm^2). Flasks were kept in incubators providing 37°C and 5% CO_2. Cellpassage was performed every 3 days. Adherent cells were released from monolayer by adding Trypsin-EDTA for 3 to 5 minutes and subcultures in the ratio described in chapter 4.1.

For long-term storage, adherent cell lines were counted with the Neubauer counting chamber. 10^6 cells per ml medium were suspended in 1ml FCS and 10% dimethyl sulphoxid (DMSO), a cryoprotective agent. Cells were stored in cryotubes at -196°C. For recovery cells were thawed swiftly in a water bath holding a temperature of 37°C and resuspended in 10ml RPMI medium with 20% FCS, 1% Glutamin and 1% Penicillin. All cells were kept on antibiotics in culture flasks for 1-2 days after recovery, but maintained and applied in experiment only on RPMI medium 1% Glutamine and 10% FCS for a consecutive period of up to 2 months.

5.2 In-vitro assays

5.2.1 Stimulation with TRAIL

The human neuroblastoma cell line KELLY was stimulated with soluble TRAIL. KELLY cells were seeded at 10 x 10^4 cells per ml medium in100µl well plates and incubated at 37°C for 24h to allow attachment and to reach a well coverage of at least 10% prior to stimulation with TRAIL. After 24h adherent cells were replenished with 200µl of fresh medium and stimulated with TRAIL at concentrations of 1, 10 and 40 ng/ml for another 24h to 48h. Experiments were performed fourfold in parallel to compensate for intra-assay variations.

Methods

5.2.2 Transient transfection

Adherent human cell lines were transiently transfected with small interfering RNAs (siRNA) (table 4.2). Small interfering RNAs were used to downregulate endogenous TRAIL on RNA and Protein level. To successfully transfect siRNAs into human cell lines liposome forming substances, such as Lipofectamine 2000 and RNAimax were used. Lipofectamine and RNAimax form liposomes which react with siRNA to complexes. These complexes fuse with cell membranes and allow cellular siRNA uptake.

For this purpose cell lines were seeded in 24-well plates and incubated at 37°C at different durations to reach a confluency of at least 5-10% at the time of transfection. For each transfection sample 1µl of transfection agent and 1µl of 20µM RNAi (20pmol) were separately diluted in 50µl of Opti-mem and mixed gently. Diluted transfection agent and diluted RNAi were combined gently. After the initial incubation time cells were replenished with 400 µl fresh growth medium and RNAi- Lipofectamine complex was added to give a final volume of 500µl. Plates were gently rocked back and forth to assure even distribution and placed at 37°C for incubation. The duration of incubation varied among the different cell lines. Transfection experiments were performed fourfold to compensate for intra-assay variation.

Cell line	HEK	MELANOMA	KELLY	SHEP
Seeding cells/ml	60.000	80.000	25.000	50.000
Incubation (h)	12	24	36	24
Agent	Lipo 2000	RNAimax	Lipo 2000	Lipo 2000
Transfection (h)	24	48	48	48
Source	A	B	C	A

Tab. 1 Transfection protocol of cell lines used in this work.
A Manufactor's protocol (Invitrogen), B (Besch *et al.*, 2009), C (Kroll,Lisa; 2012)

Methods

5.2.3 Caspase inhibition

The human neuroblastoma cell line KELLY was subjected to caspase inhibition with the pan-caspase inhibitor Q-VD prior to being transiently transfected with TRAIL targeting siRNA. Q-VD [N-(2-Quinolyl)valyl-aspartly-(2,6-difluorophenoxy)methyl Ketone] irreversibly binds caspases (Caserta *et al.*, 2003). For caspase inhibition cells were seeded in 24-well plates and pan-caspase inhibitor Q-VD was added 1 h prior to transfection to reach an end-concentration of 50µM. Q-VD was repeatedly added after 48h. Control samples were treated with the Q-VD solvent DMSO alone.

5.3 Cell growth analysis using CellScreen

Cell growth analysis was carried out with the use of CellScreen. CellScreen is a computer supported microscope which consists of an inverse microscope with 10x and 4x magnification, a CCD- Camera (1024x1024 Pixel), a motorized plate table and a high power processor. CellScreen takes pictures of exactly the same cell in culture over time without disturbing culture conditions. Adherent cells of the present work were acquired in the AC mode with 4x magnification. The percentage of cell coverage was estimated by automated analysis of each picture using the PA adhesion software (Innovatis). Growth curves were calculated from the collected data. Cell growth analysis was performed following TRAIL stimulation (see chapter 5.2.1) and transient transfection (see chapter 5.2.2).

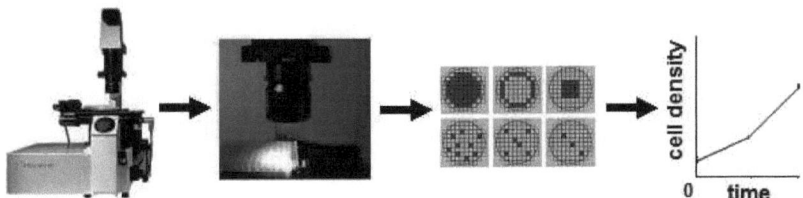

Figure 2. Cell growth analysis using CellScreen.
CellScreen, an automated microscope, measured the cell coverage (cell density) of preselected wells at defined time points. Growth curves were calculated from these data.

Methods

5.4 Cell death analysis using Fluorescence activated cell sorting (FACS)

Cell death analysis was carried out using Fluorescence activated cell sorting (FACS). By means of flow cytometric analysis different cell populations were characterized according to cellular size, granularity or by the attachment of fluorescent dye or fluorescent labeled antibodies. Adherent cells entering cell death are characterized by a decreased content of DNA due to DNA fragmentation and a consecutive loss of nuclear DNA. Specific DNA labeling agents, such as the fluorescent DNA intercalating agent Propidium Iodide (PI), attach to fragmented intracellular DNA of apoptotic cells and emit light upon laser beam stimulation (Nicoletti *et al.*, 1991). Light detectors measure the light emission of a specific wavelength and allow the detection of cells entering cell death.

To analyze cell death adherent cells were pelleted and lysated with Nicoletti buffer at 4°C for 30 minutes to allow cell membrane degradation. Following the incubation period cells were stained with Propidium Iodide (PI) (50 μg/ml). PI emits a fluorescent light at an emission maximum of 617nm. Fluorescence intensity of cells pre-treated with PI was measured by flow cytometry in channel FL-3 (Emission fluorescence wavelength (λ) = 650nm). Acquired data were analyzed using Cell Quest Pro Software (BD Bioscience, USA) to determine absolute cell death rates.

Figure 3 illustrates flow cytometric analysis of adherent cells entering cell death which were characterized by a lower DNA content and therefore lower detected fluorescence intensity (M_1).

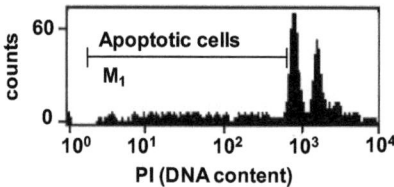

Figure 3. Analysis of apoptosis in adherent cells using FACS.
Cells were subjected to lysis with Nicoletti buffer and stained with Propidium Iodide (PI) to visualize DNA content. Cells with low DNA content (M_1) represent apoptotic cell fraction.

Methods

5.5 Analysis of transfection efficiency using Fluorescence activated cell sorting (FACS)

Cellular detection of siRNA after transient transfection was performed using flow cytometric analysis. Cellular delivery of siRNA is a significant factor for successful downregulation of proteins (Elbashir *et al.*, 2001; Ovcharenko *et al.*, 2005). To assess successful delivery of siRNA cells were transfected with Fluorochrom-labeled siRNAs (FAM-labeled control siRNA, FAM-labeled TRAIL targeting siRNA) and subjected to flow cytometric analysis. FAM-labeled siRNAs are dye conjugated oligonucleotides which emit light at a maximum emission wave length (λ) of 520nm when stimulated.

To estimate the amount of successfully transfected cells with FAM-labeled siRNAs, cells were detached from cell plates after transient transfection using Trypsin. Enzymatic activity of Trypsin was stopped by the addition of culture medium. Cell suspension was transferred in 1ml eppendorf tubes and subjected to two washing steps with PBS. 250µl of cell suspension were analyzed for fluorescence intensity using flow cytometry. Fluorescence of stimulated cells was detected by light detectors of flow cytometry using channel FL-1 (Emission fluorescence wavelength (λ) = 530nm). Acquired data were analyzed using Cell Quest Pro Software (BD Bioscience, USA).

5.6 Statistical Analysis

To determine statistical significance of results the unpaired ANOVA-Test (one-way analysis of variance) was applied. Statistical significance was determined by p-values < 0.05, respectively < 0.01 (highly significant), and was indicated in the present work by * respectively **.

Methods

5.7 RNA/DNA studies

5.7.1 RNA Isolation and quantification

RNA was isolated from cultured cells using the SV total RNA Isolation System (Promega). Approximately 10^6 cells were collected and pelleted to receive a sufficient RNA yield. All steps of cell lysation and RNA isolation were carried out according to manufactor´s protocol. Total isolated RNA was quantified and quality of RNA estimated using the UV spectrophotometer Nanodrop-ND 2000 (Thermoscientific, Bonn).

For the purpose of quantification 1-2 µl of an undiluted solution sample were pipetted on a measuring pedestal to assess light absorbance of a specific wavelength. In a concentration dependent manner UV spectrometer detected the absorption of light of a solution containing nucleic acid. The concentration of single stranded nucleic acid was estimated in reference to the Beer-Lambert equation by measuring the absorption of light at a wavelength of 260nm and 280nm (A_{260}/A_{280}) (Kallansrud and Ward, 1996). The quality of isolated RNA was estimated calculating the ratio of light absorption at a wavelength of 260 and 230nm (A_{260}/A_{230}). By this means contamination, for instance protein or phenol, were excluded. According to the manufactor´s protocol RNA with the following absorbance ratio was considered to be free of contaminants and applied in experiments of the present work:

$$A_{260}/A_{280}: 1.8 - 2.0, A_{260}/A_{230}: 1.8 - 2.2$$

5.7.2 Reverse Transcriptase Reaction

Isolated total RNA was subjected to Reverse Transcription Reaction after determining the concentration and purity of total RNA. Reverse Transcriptase Reaction, using the High Capacity cDNA Reverse Transcription kit (Applied Biosystems), allows the conversion of RNA strands to complementary DNA (cDNA). Reverse Transcriptase Reaction was performed with the aim to quantify levels of mRNA expression in different cell lines and validate the down regulating potential of various TRAIL targeting siRNAs.

To synthesize single-stranded cDNA from total RNA up to 2 µg of isolated RNA were applied in a 20 µl reaction. Amounts greater than 2 µg were not used due to an inhibitory effect. RNA and kit components were thawed on ice. Reverse Transcriptase mastermix consisting of 2 µl 10x RT Buffer, 0.8 µl 25x dNTP Mix (100mM), 2 µl 10x RT Random Primers and 1 µl of reverse Transcriptase were prepared for a 20 µl reaction. RNA, equaling an amount of 2 µg,

Methods

and RNAse free H$_2$0 were added to the mixture and content was centrifuged briefly to eliminate air bubbles. Reaction tubes were loaded into the thermal cycler and initially incubated for 10 minutes at 25°C and subsequently for 120 min at 37°C. The reaction was terminated by increasing the temperature to 85°C for 5 seconds. Synthesized cDNA was stored at -20°C or directly used as a template for qRT-PCR.

5.7.3 Quantitative Real-Time Polymerase Chain Reaction (qRT-PCR)

To quantify synthesized cDNA in the present work quantitive Real-Time Polymerase Chain reaction (qRT-PCR) was performed using Lightcycler (Roche Diagnostics, Mannheim). QRT-PCR is based on general principles of Polymerase Chain reaction for the qualitative detection of DNA and additionally measures fluorescence in real-time for its quantification. The detection of TRAIL DNA by qRT-PCR using LightCycler was optimized in previous work of our research lab (Kroll, Lisa; 2012).

The detection of specific DNA sequences is realized using pairs of short oligonucleotides (primers) which are complementary to a segment of the DNA of interest. In a PCR cycle a temperature increase is initially generated to separate double stranded DNA into two single strands (denaturation). A subsequent decrease in temperature allows the attachment of primers to the DNA sequence of interest (annealing). The addition of a thermo-stable DNA polymerase (Taq Polymerase) initiates the amplification of the DNA sequence of interest (extension) and a complimentary copy of the template DNA is generated. The PCR cycle (denaturation, annealing, extention) repeats itself, as copies of generated DNA serve as templates.

The quantification of DNA is realized by the application of a DNA binding dye, SYBR Green, during the PCR process. SYBR green, a fluorescent dye, binds to double stranded DNA in a concentration dependent manner. Upon binding light of a different wavelength is emitted and the intensity of fluorescence is analyzed.

For LightCycler reaction a mastermix containing 2 μl light cycler mix (Roche), 0.5 μl forward primer, 0.5 μl reverse primer, 6 μl water was prepared. Reagents were mixed within a PCR workstation to avoid contamination with DNA. 9 μl of LightCycler mastermix were filled in LightCycler glass capillaries and 1 μl of cDNA was added as PCR template. Samples were pipetted in duplicates to eliminate pipetting errors. These steps were performed outside the

Methods

PCR workstation. As a next step capillaries were closed, centrifuged and placed into the LightCycler roter. For the quantification of TRAIL qRT-PCR using LightCycler was performed with temperature targets listed in table 2.

Program	Temperature and time
Denaturation	95°C for 10 min
Amplification	
- Denaturation	95°C for 2s
- Annealing	61°C for 18s
- Elongation	72°C for 15s
Melting curve analysis	
- 1. part	65°C for 15 s
- 2. part	65°C - 95°C, slope 0.1 °C/s
Cooling of instrument	40°C for 10s

*Number of cycles: 45

Tab. 2. **Temperature targets for RT-PCR using LightCycler (Roche diagnostics, Mannheim).**
Protocol was optimized in previous work of our research laboratory (Kroll, Lisa; 2012).

5.7.4 Analysis of qRT-PCR (crossing point and melting curve analysis)

Fluorescence measured with qRT-PCR was analyzed using the LightCycler software version 4.05. By means of fluorescence analysis the quality and quantity of amplified DNA was measured.

For quality purposes melting curve analysis was performed. During qRT-PCR melting curves are generated to measure the quality of the amplified DNA product. A slow temperature increase (65°C to 95° at 0.1°C per s, see Table.2.) is generated for this purpose. Amplified DNA has a characteristic melting temperature (T_M). Once the specific melting temperature is reached, DNA denaturizes and the fluorescence signal terminates, as SYBR-green loses its binding site. Hereby melting curves are generated which allow the analysis of the specificity of amplified DNA products. Identical PCR products have identical melting temperatures and

Methods

were applied in further analysis. Primer mismatches, which do not influence DNA product quantification, have a very low melting temperature and can thus be identified. PCR products contaminated with by-products, are identified by multiple melting temperatures during a single analysis, and are thus excluded from further analysis. Figure 4 illustrates melting curves for the TRAIL product as generated by the light cycler software 4.05.

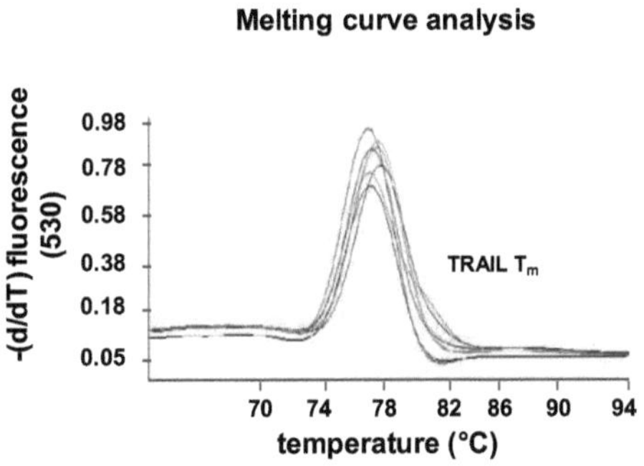

Melting curve analysis

[Chart: -(d/dT) fluorescence (530) vs temperature (°C), showing TRAIL T_m peak around 82°C]

Figure 4. Overlapping melting temperatures indicate a high specificity of the PCR-product TRAIL.
Melting curve of the PCR product TRAIL was generated to test for specificity of the amplified product. For this purpose the melting temperature was calculated (T_m). To facilitate the read-out the first derivative of fluorescence was charted against temperature.

For quantification purposes Crossing Point (CP) analysis was performed. By means of CP analysis the amount of amplified DNA was estimated by measuring fluorescence intensity. A threshold for fluorescence detection was set and cycle numbers were measured when threshold levels were reached (CP value). High amplification cycles are required to reach threshold levels for the detection of fluorescence in samples with low initial concentration of target DNA. In the presenting work mRNA transcripts of TRAIL were relatively quantified to allow standardization of results using the non- regulated housekeeper gene Hypoxanthin-Guanin-Phosphoribosyltransferase (HPRT) as a reference gene.

Methods

To quantify the relative amount of the DNA of interest, and respectively the amount of RNA of interest, CP values were measured of TRAIL and HPRT and applied in the following mathematical model (Pfaffl, 2001):

$$\text{Relative mRNA transcripts} = \frac{(E_{TRAIL})^{\Delta CP\ TRAIL\ (control-sample)}}{(E_{HPRT})^{\Delta CP\ HPRT\ (control-sample)}}$$

Figure 5. Mathematical model for relative quantification of endogenous TRAIL mRNA applying crossing point values.
E_{TRAIL} = Efficiency of TRAIL primer = 1.88, E_{HPRT} = efficiency of HPRT Primer = 1.96.

5.8 Protein studies

5.8.1 Cell lysis

To measure protein expression of endogenous TRAIL cultured cells were subjected to cell lysis and subsequent gel electrophoresis and immunoblotting.

2.5×10^5 HEK cells were seeded in 6 well plates and cultured at 37°C for 24h to 72h. Well plates were transferred from the incubator on ice to carry out steps of cell lysis. Growth medium was removed and cells were washed with 1ml of PBS (4°C). 200μl of cytoplasmatic lysis buffer (SDS Sample Buffer) were supplemented with Protease inhibitor (1%) and added to well plates. A cell scraper was used to efficiently detach cells from well plates and assist in cell lysis. The generated cell lysates was transferred to pre-labeled Eppendorf-tubes and stored at -20°C.

Prior to gel electrophoresis and immunoblotting cell lysates were treated with ultrasound, at an amplitude of 10% and 5 (20) impulses, heated for 5 minutes at 95°C and vortexed briefly. These steps assisted in decreasing lysates' viscosity and in protein denaturation. Cell lysate were then loaded onto a SDS-Polyacrylamide gel.

Methods

5.8.2 SDS-Polyacrylamid Gel Electrophoresis (PAGE)

SDS-Polyacrylamid Gel electrophoresis describes a method in which denatured proteins are separated into subunits according to size while migrating through the pores of a gel matrix in response to an electric field. Different proteins of same molecular weight migrate through the gel in a similar pace. To separate endogenous TRAIL from other proteins and subsequently measure protein's expression level, cell lysates were subjected to SDS-Polyacrylamide Gel Electrophoresis.

SDS-Polyacrylamide gel consisted of a stacking gel and a running gel. Acrylamide concentration determines the size of the pores of the gel and thus the degree of protein resolution. The following acrylamide concentration and gel composition was chosen to identify endogenous TRAIL (35kB):

Stacking gel (5%):	680 µL	ddH$_2$O
	170 µL	Acrylamide (30%)
	130 µL	Puffer B
	10 µL	SDS (20%)
	10 µL	APS (10%)
Running Gel (12%):	1.6 mL	ddH$_2$O
	2 mL	Acrylamide (30%)
	1.25 mL	Puffer A
	50 µL	SDS (20%)
	50 µL	APS (10%)
	2 µL	TEMED

The prepared polyacrylamide gel was overlaid with running buffer. 25µl of cell lysate and 2 µl of a standardized protein ladder (rainbowmarker) were loaded into the pockets of the stacking gel. Running buffer was added to the cover gel creating a close circuit. Gel was subjected for the initial 30 minutes to a voltage of 80 V to allow protein transfer into the running gel and then subjected for the following 180 minutes to a voltage of 180 V to allow protein separation.

5.8.3 Immunoblotting and Immunodetection

Immunoblot and immunodetection are analytical methods which are used to detect proteins separated by SDS-PAGE. As a first step proteins are transferred onto a Polyvinylidene difluoride (PVDF) membrane to make proteins accessible to antibody detection (immunoblot). As a second step PVDF membrane is subjected to protein specific antibodies (immunodetection).

2 Whatman-papers were soaked in transfer buffer and instilled into the blotting chamber (Trans-Blot SD Semi-dry transfer cell). The PVDF membrane was activated in Methanol for 1 minute, shortly washed with transfer buffer and placed onto Whatman-papers. The protein carrying SDS-gel was washed with transfer buffer and placed onto the PVDF membrane. As the contact between membrane and gel is critical for protein transfer air bubbles were avoided. Finally, 2 Whatman papers soaked with transfer buffer were placed onto the SDS-gel. The blotting chamber was subjected to an electrical field of 200 mA for 120min to allow protein transfer.

In preparation for immunodetection PVDF membrane was incubated at room temperature for 1 hour in TBST with 5 % powdered milk. This step was taken to prevent all non-specific binding of antibodies with the PVDF membrane. After blocking the PVDF membrane was incubated overnight with a diluted solution of antigen specific antibody (primary antibody) at 4°C. 3 x 15 minute washing steps with TBST followed. For primary antibody detection and signal enhancement PVDF membrane was incubated with species specific antibodies (secondary antibodies) for 1 hour at room temperature (see chapter 4.3). Three additional 10 minute washing steps with TBST followed. Immunodetection was carried out using the chemo-luminescence reaction. Secondary antibodies were linked to the enzyme horseradish peroxidase (HRP), which produced luminescence when used in conjunction with a chemo luminescent agent (ECL). 1 ml of ECL was applied for 1 minute to the PVDF membrane. The PVDF membrane was placed into an x-ray film cassette. Exposure time ranged from 3 minutes for the detection of Anti-Trail Antibody (Peprotech) to 1 second for the detection of Anti-GAPDH Antibody (Affinity Bioreagents).

6 Results

The importance of soluble and endogenous TRAIL in tumor biology has been shown for TRAIL sensitive cancers. Data provided evidence that the upregulation of endogenous TRAIL in apoptosis sensitive cancers increased cancer immune surveillance and thus suppressed cancer cell growth (Takeda et al., 2002; Sanlioglu et al., 2008). In the past studies have shown that a variety of cancers were resistant to TRAIL induced cell death and report TRAIL mediated survival and proliferation as a new adverse effect of TRAIL in cancer therapy (Baader et al., 2005). To investigate the potential role of endogenous TRAIL as an endogenous growth factor in a subgroup of TRAIL resistant cancers the present work examined the effect of the downregulation of endogenous TRAIL on spontaneous cell growth in different human cancer cell lines, and in particular in the neuroblastoma cell line KELLY, a cell line sensitive to TRAIL mediated proliferation.

6.1 TRAIL mediated proliferation

Our research group has previously described TRAIL mediated survival and proliferation as an adverse effect of cancer therapy on primary leukemia cells and furthermore on the human neuroblastoma cell line KELLY (Baader et al., 2005). At the beginning of my investigation I examined whether I could reproduce TRAIL mediated proliferation on the neuroblastoma cell line KELLY in the experimental setting applied. In this case KELLY cells would serve as an adequate cell line to study the function of endogenous TRAIL.

KELLY cells were cultured in well plates and incubated with TRAIL at various concentrations (1, 10 or 40 ng/ml) for 48h. To evaluate cell growth the density of cultured cells were measured using CellScreen. CellScreen, an automated microscope which takes pictures of exactly the same cell in culture over time, estimated the percentage of well coverage by an automated analysis of each picture and calculated the cell density (cell numbers per cm^2) using a standard curve. From this data growth curves were generated. Figure 6 illustrates the results of TRAIL stimulation of the neuroblastoma cell line KELLY.

Results

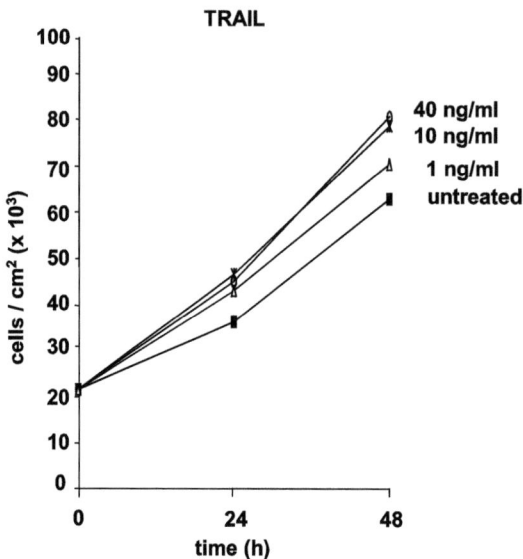

Figure 6. TRAIL mediated increase in cell density of the neuroblastoma cell line KELLY.
KELLY cells were stimulated with 1, 10 or 40 ng/ml TRAIL and incubated for 48h. Untreated KELLY cells were used as control. Cell density was measured using CellScreen at 0h, 24h and 48h. One representative of two independent experiments is shown.

The data of the present study showed an increase of density in TRAIL treated cells in culture at 24h and 48h in comparison to untreated control cells. The strongest increase in growth of TRAIL stimulated cells took place in the first 24h. Furthermore growth increase was concentration dependent, as treatment with 10 ng/ml and 40ng/ml of TRAIL lead to a greater increase within the first 24h than treatment with 1 ng/ml TRAIL. Thus, the data of the present work showed that KELLY cells responded to TRAIL treatment with an increase of cell density, which is a strong indicator of cell growth and cell proliferation. Taken together the initial experiments confirmed the presence of TRAIL mediated proliferation on the neuroblastoma cells line KELLY, as initially described by my research group (Baader et al., 2005). The results of the present study thus emphasize the suitability of the human neuroblastoma cell line KELLY to be applied in the present study in order to investigate the role of endogenous TRAIL as a growth promoting factor.

Results

6.2 Downregulation of endogenous TRAIL: optimization

After showing that the human neuroblastoma cell line KELLY proliferates when treated with TRAIL, the downregulation of endogenous TRAIL using TRAIL targeting interfering RNA was optimized. In a first step various cell lines were screened for endogenous TRAIL expression to determine the optimal cell line for the downregulation of TRAIL. In a second step fluorescent dye-labeled siRNAs were transfected into selected cells to evaluate the delivery of siRNA, as siRNA-based gene delivery is a significant factor for downregulation (Ovcharenko *et al.*, 2005). As a last step various siRNAs were examined for their efficiency to downregulate endogenous TRAIL on mRNA and protein level.

6.2.1 Screening human cell lines for endogenous TRAIL expression

Studies showed that endogenous TRAIL expression varies considerably throughout the tissue (Spierings *et al.*, 2004). Furthermore it has been shown that cultured cells up- or downregulate endogenous TRAIL production according to their activation status (Ehrlich *et al.*, 2003). As an abundant production of target protein facilitates the detection of an efficient downregulation by means of RNA interference, various human cancer cell lines were screened for high endogenous TRAIL expression. Human cell lines were screened by measuring RNA expression of endogenous TRAIL with Real-time Polymerase Chain Reaction (RT-PCR). RT-PCR was optimized for the detection and quantification of endogenous TRAIL in previous work of our research laboratory (Kroll, 2011).

For this purpose multiple human cancer cell lines were thawed and kept in culture for 7 days. All cells were held in optimal culture conditions without usage of antibiotics before being prepared for RT-PCR. TRAIL overexpressing HEK cells, HEK-TRAIL, a cell line which was stably transfected with a constitutively TRAIL expressing vector in our research lab, served as a positive control. Furthermore, a melanoma cell line (MEL) was stimulated with Polyinosinic Polycytidylic acid (Poly I:C), a short double stranded RNA which has been shown to have an immunostimulatory potential (Alexopoulou *et al.*, 2001). As immunostimulators are strong up-regulators of endogenous TRAIL expression (Bretz *et al.*, 1999), I expected to measure high endogenous TRAIL production in POLY (I:C) stimulated cell lines.

Results

For RT-PCR cultured cell lines were harvested and total RNA extracted. Total extracted RNA was quantified and subjected to reverse transcription. For the quantification of TRAIL DNA, HPRT, a housekeeper gene, was simultaneously detected and used as a reference for the expression of endogenous TRAIL (relative mRNA transcripts). Housekeeper genes are stably expressed genes which are not influenced by experimental settings. Figure 7 illustrates the results of the present study showing relative expression levels of TRAIL mRNA in selected cell lines.

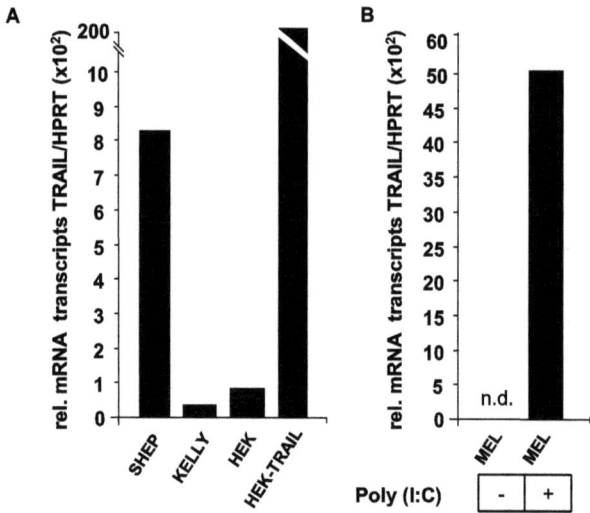

Figure 7. A. Variability of endogenous TRAIL expression on mRNA level in human cell lines. Selected human cell lines were cultured and subjected to RNA isolation and mRNA measurement using RT-PCR. Illustrated are mRNA levels of endogenous TRAIL expression in relation to the expression of the housekeeper gene, HPRT (rel. mRNA transcripts). **B. Up-regulation of endogenous TRAIL expression on mRNA level by Poly (I:C).** Melanoma cells (Mel) were subjected to the stimulation with the synthetic RNA analog, Poly (I:C), for 17h (+), or left unstimulated (-). Thereafter cells were subjected to RNA isolation and mRNA measurement using RT-PCR. Illustrated are mRNA levels of endogenous TRAIL expression in relation to the housekeeper gene, HPRT (rel. mRNA transcripts). n.d.=not detected.

Results

The results demonstrated that throughout the cell lines a considerable difference of endogenous TRAIL expression existed (figure 7 A). Untreated cells showed low levels of endogenous TRAIL production in comparison to TRAIL over-expressing HEK cells, which served as a positive control. The selected neuroblastoma cell line Kelly expressed the lowest amounts of endogenous TRAIL. Furthermore, unstimulated Melanoma cells proved to be natively deficient of endogenous TRAIL, as endogenous TRAIL was not detected using RT-PCR (figure 7 B). Poly (I:C) stimulated Melanoma cells in contrast showed an upregulation of endogenous TRAIL on RNA level. A melting curve analysis validated the purity and thus the accuracy of the quantification data (see chapter 5.7.3).

Taken together, with this data I showed that endogenous TRAIL expression is highly variable throughout human cancer cell lines. As all cells were kept in similar culture conditions, I interpreted differences of endogenous TRAIL expression as a result of variable endogenous production. As Kelly cells produced a very little amount of endogenous TRAIL, they were considered not to be suitable for optimization experiments. For the same reason non-stimulated Melanoma cells proved to be unsuitable. Furthermore, the data of the present study confirmed that immunostimulators, such as Poly (I:C), upregulated endogenous TRAIL production on RNA level. Therefore, Poly (I:C) stimulated Melanoma cells and the TRAIL over-expressing control cell line, HEK-TRAIL, were selected for the following optimization experiments.

6.2.2 Evaluation of siRNA delivery

As a next step siRNA delivery was evaluated. Cellular delivery of siRNA is a significant factor for successful downregulation of gene products of interest (Elbashir *et al.*, 2001; Ovcharenko *et al.*, 2005). To assess successful delivery of siRNA cells were transfected with FAM-labeled control siRNAs and subjected to flow cytometric analysis. FAM-labeled siRNAs are fluorencent-dye labeled oligonucleotides which are used to trace transfected cells.

Results

Both endogenous TRAIL over-expressing HEK cells, HEK-TRAIL, and Melanoma cells were transfected according to published transfection protocol using liposome forming substances (see chapter 5.2.1). Melanoma cells were incubated with FAM-labeled siRNA for 48h and retransfected for another 17h while simultaneously being stimulated with Poly (I:C). HEK-TRAIL cells were incubated with Fam-labeled siRNA for 24h. Cells treated with transfection medium without siRNA (mock transfection) were used as controls. Fluorescence was measured in channel FL-1, which was termed FAM, using flow cytometry. Figure 8 shows a representative result of flow cytometric analysis of treated cells.

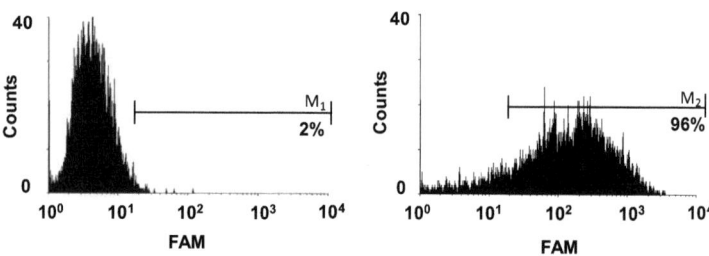

Figure 8. Successful cell delivery of FAM-labeled siRNA.
Melanoma and HEK cells were transfected with FAM-labeled control siRNA according to transfection protocol and subjected to flow cytometric analysis. The illustration shows histograms created by flow cytometric analysis of HEK cells which were transfected with FAM-labeled control siRNA. Fluorescence intensity is plotted against the number of measured cells (counts). The histogram on the left shows a cell sample subjected to mock transfection (no siRNA). The histogram on the right shows a cell sample transfected with FAM-labeled siRNA. M_2 delineates transfected cell fraction.

Flow cytometry analysis rendered histograms which showed a marked right shift of fluorescence intensity in cells treated with transfection medium and siRNA. The right shifted histogram represented an increase in fluorescence intensity and thus indicated a high number of successfully transfected cells. A successful siRNA delivery was detected in 94% ($M_2 - M_1$) of HEK-TRAIL cells. Same transfection results were achieved in Melanoma cells (data not shown). These results confirmed the successful delivery of siRNA by means of transfection protocols used in the present study.

Results

6.2.3 Evaluation of siRNA efficiency

In a last step of optimization I examined various siRNAs for their efficiency to down-regulate endogenous TRAIL on mRNA and protein level. The aim of this undertaking was to find a powerful tool of downregulation in order to study the function of endogenous TRAIL.

6.2.3.1 Efficiency on RNA level

In an initial step the efficiency of several TRAIL targeting siRNAs on RNA level was evaluated. The aim of this undertaking was to identify an efficient siRNA which suppressed endogenous TRAIL on RNA level and which would be used to study the role of endogenous TRAIL. For this purpose I selected three promising siRNAs, whose sequences met published guidelines for efficient inhibition (Ui-Tei *et al.*, 2007). I transfected cells with TRAIL targeting siRNAs and assessed siRNA delivery using flow cytometry as previously described (see chapter 6.2.2). Cells were subjected to measurement of RNA only if transfection rates of 90% and above were reached. Down-regulation of endogenous TRAIL was evaluated on RNA level using RT-PCR. For this purpose Poly (I:C) stimulated melanoma cells, which proved to have a high endogenous TRAIL expression in previous experiments, were used.

Poly (I:C) stimulated melanoma cells were transfected according to transfection protocol with three different TRAIL targeting siRNAs. Control cells were either transfected with control siRNA and stimulated with Poly (I:C) (co), or left non-transfected and non-stimulated (-). 17h after retransfection and restimulation cells were harvested for RNA isolation. RNA expression of TRAIL was quantified using RT-PCR.

Results

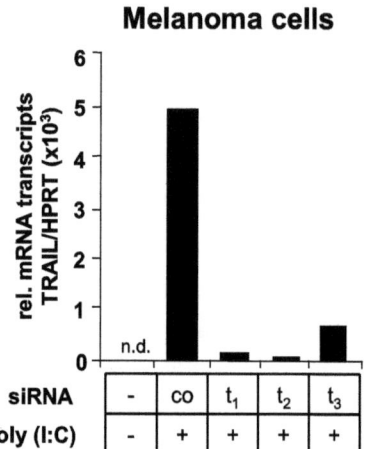

Figure 9. Efficient downregulation of endogenous TRAIL on mRNA level by three different TRAIL targeting siRNAs.
Melanoma cells were stimulated with Poly (I:C) and transfected with three TRAIL targeting siRNAs (t_1, t_2, t_3) or control siRNA (co) for 48h. Unstimulated and untransfected cells served as control. Afterwards cells were subjected to RNA isolation and mRNA measurement using RT-PCR. Shown are expression levels of endogenous TRAIL mRNA in relation to the housekeeper gene, HPRT (rel. mRNA transcripts).

The results of the present experiment, illustrated in figure 9, showed a significant decrease of TRAIL expression in melanoma cells, treated with TRAIL targeting siRNAs (siTRAIL t_1, t_2, t_3). Among the three siRNAs tested TRAIL targeting siRNA t_2 was identified as the most effective siRNA, inhibiting TRAIL RNA production by 99% in comparison to non-silencing control siRNA (co). SiRNA t_1 showed a slightly lower TRAIL reducing potential on RNA level. Poly (I:C) stimulated melanoma cells transfected with non-silencing siRNA in contrast showed high levels of endogenous TRAIL expression. Non-transfected and non-stimulated melanoma cells again demonstrated no detectable endogenous TRAIL production. A melting curve analysis validated the purity and thus the accuracy of the quantification data (not shown).

Results

6.2.3.2 Efficiency on Protein Level

In a next step I tested the efficiency of the selected siRNA on protein level. Studies had shown that the downregulation on mRNA level must not extend to the protein level, especially in proteins with a low turn-over rate (Dykxhoorn et al., 2003; Wu et al., 2004). To prove that TRAIL targeting siRNA t_2 downregulated TRAIL on protein level, endogenous TRAIL expression of siRNA t_2 transfected cells was evaluated using western blot. For this purpose the TRAIL over-expressing human cell line, HEK-TRAIL, was applied.

TRAIL over-expressing HEK cells, HEK-TRAIL, were transfected for 24h with siRNA t_2 and control siRNA and by means of western blot analysis endogenous TRAIL production was measured. Endogenous TRAIL production was directly measured at the end of transfection (24h) and every 12h thereafter (32h, 48h, 72h) to evaluate the duration of downregulation. Cells were subjected to flow cytometric analysis to assure adequate siRNA delivery prior to western blot analysis. Only cells with transfection rates of 90% and above were subjected to Western blot analysis. GAPDH, a constitutively expressed house keeper protein, was measured alongside of TRAIL to function as a reference for the quantification of endogenous TRAIL. Figure 10 shows the results of the western blot analysis.

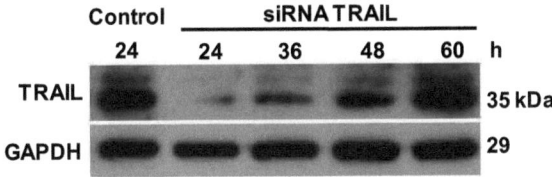

Figure 10. Efficent downregulation of endogenous TRAIL on protein level by TRAIL targeting siRNA.
HEK cells overexpressing TRAIL (HEK-TRAIL) were treated for 24h with control siRNA (control) and TRAIL targeting siRNA (siRNA TRAIL). Transfected cells were harvested for lysis directly after transfection at 24h and after an additional treatment free period at 36, 48 and 60h. Shown are results of western blot analysis for endogenous TRAIL. GAPDH served as a loading control.

Results

The results of the western blot analysis confirmed the potential of siRNA t_2 to downregulate endogenous TRAIL on protein level. The results of the present study showed that cells transfected with TRAIL targeting siRNA produced lower levels of endogenous TRAIL on protein level than cells transfected with non-silencing siRNA (control). A marked reduction of protein production was observed at 24h and 32 h after start of transfection. At 48h and thereafter efficacy of protein inhibition was reduced and reversed at 72h as seen by the reaccumulation of TRAIL protein to control conditions (72h). GAPDH was detected in equal amounts throughout the samples.

Taken together, the present study showed that TRAIL targeting siRNA t_2 had a greater potential to downregulate endogenous TRAIL on mRNA level than other TRAIL targeting siRNAs tested and moreover had an inhibitory potential on protein level.

In summary, the experiments of the present study showed that TRAIL targeting siRNA can be successfully delivered into Poly (I:C) stimulated Melanoma cells and TRAIL over-expressing HEK cell, two cell lines which showed very high endogenous TRAIL expression. Transfection efficiencies of 90% and above were attained in cells treated with siRNA. Downregulation studies with various TRAIL targeting siRNAs showed the highest inhibiting potential of TRAIL targeting siRNA t_2 on RNA and protein level. Furthermore, inhibition of endogenous TRAIL was not cell line specific. Therefore, the present studies showed that TRAIL targeting siRNA t_2 served as a powerful tool to study the function of endogenous TRAIL.

6.3 Downregulation of endogenous TRAIL: screening for effects on cell growth

In a subpopulation of TRAIL resistant cancer cells TRAIL mediated cancer cell growth (Baader *et al.*, 2005). In the following study the growth promoting potential of endogenous TRAIL in tumor cells showing TRAIL mediated proliferation is investigated.

For this purpose human cancer cell lines were transfected with TRAIL targeting siRNA t_2, which in previous studies had shown a strong potential to downregulate endogenous TRAIL. Thereafter, human cell lines were screened for effects on cell growth using CellScreen. Downregulation studies were carried out on two human cell lines showing sensitivity to TRAIL mediated apoptosis, SHEP cells (Baader *et al.*, 2005) and HEK cells (Shetty *et al.*, 2002) and one cell line showing sensitivity to TRAIL mediated proliferation, the human neuroblastoma

Results

cell lines KELLY (Baader *et al.*, 2005). Cells were transfected according to previously described transfection protocols (see chapter 5.2.1). In reference to previous experiments of the present work which showed a transient character of downregulation during transfection (see Figure 10), transfection times of the neuroblastoma cell line SHEP and KELLY were extended from initial 24h to 48h to prolong observation time. The transfection time of HEK cells remained at 24h due to high sensitivity to the toxicity of the transfection medium. To ensure adequate siRNA delivery additional transfection with fluorescent dye-labeled siRNA t_2 with subsequent flow cytometric analysis was carried out. Analysis of siRNA delivery and analysis of cell growth of transfected HEK, SHEP and KELLY cells are illustrated in Figure 11, Figure 12 and Figure 13.

Flow cytometric analysis of transfected HEK cells confirmed a successful delivery of fluorescent dye-labeled siRNA as illustrated by a right shifted histogram. 92% ($M_2 - M_1$) of HEK cells were successfully transfected, a transfection efficiency which was consistent with previously shown studies of cells transfected with TRAIL targeting siRNA and successful downregulation of endogenous TRAIL (chapter 6.2.3.). Subsequent cell growth analysis of HEK cells using CellScreen showed similar cell growth behavior of control cells transfected with non-silencing siRNA (siRNA control) and cells transfected with TRAIL targeting siRNA (siRNA TRAIL) at 24h and 48h respectively. Both control siRNA transfected cells and TRAIL targeting siRNA transfected cells showed cell densities of approximately 45.000 cells per cm^2 at 48 h of cell growth analysis.

Similar observations were made for the human cell line SHEP as illustrated in Figure 12. 90% ($M_2 - M_1$) of SHEP cells were successfully transfected when analyzed by flow cytometry, confirming successful delivery of TRAIL targeting siRNA. SHEP cells transfected with TRAIL targeting siRNA and untransfected control cells showed no difference in cell growth for 48h of growth analysis performed by CellScreen. Both untransfected cells and TRAIL targeting siRNA transfected cells showed cell densities of approximately 70.000 cells per cm^2 at 48 h after start of transfection. SHEP cells transfected with non-silencing control siRNA showed slightly lower cell densities at 48h of growth analysis.

HEK

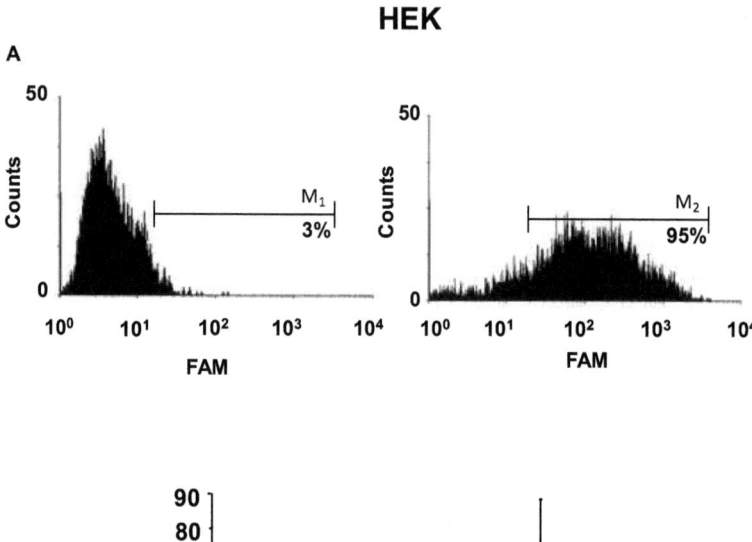

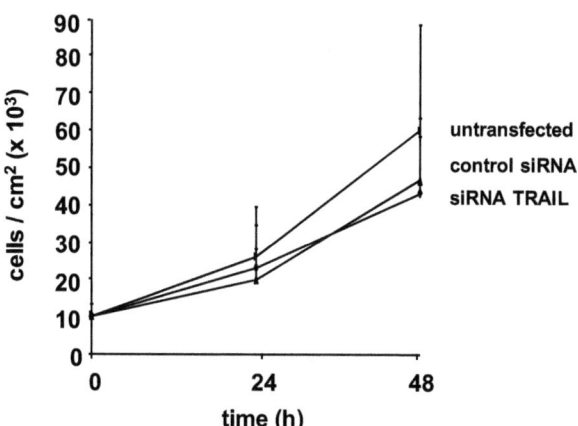

Figure 11. Transfection with TRAIL targeting siRNA shows no effect on cell growth in HEK cells.
A. HEK cells were treated for 24h with FAM-labeled TRAIL targeting siRNA (siRNA TRAIL) and subjected to flow cytometric analysis to evaluate siRNA delivery. Shown are histograms of a representative sample. M_2 delineates transfected cell fraction. **B.** HEK cells were transfected for 24h with TRAIL targeting siRNA (siRNA TRAIL) and control siRNA. Cells were subjected to CellScreen measurement for 48h to evaluate cell growth. Untransfected cells served as control. Error bars represent standard deviation of two independent experiments.

SHEP

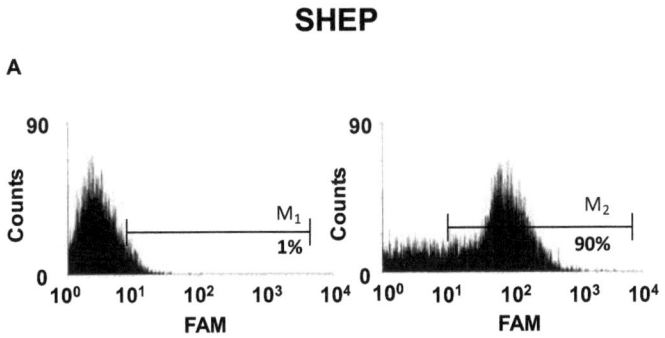

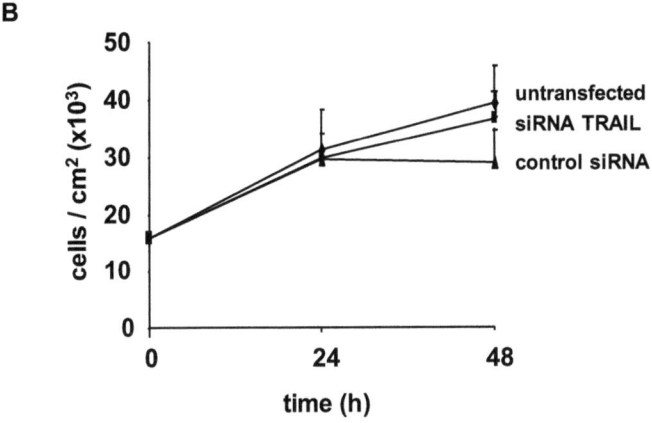

Figure 12. Transfection with TRAIL targeting siRNA shows no effect on cell growth in SHEP cells.
A. SHEP cells were treated for 48h with FAM-labeled TRAIL targeting siRNA (siRNA TRAIL) and subjected to flow cytometric analysis to evaluate siRNA delivery. Shown are histograms of a representative sample with M_2 delineating transfected cell fraction. **B.** SHEP cells were transfected for 48h with TRAIL targeting siRNA (siRNA TRAIL) and control siRNA and afterwards subjected to cell growth analysis using CellScreen. Untransfected cells served as control. Error bars represent standard deviation of two independent experiments.

Results

As a next step the human neuroblastoma cell line KELLY, a cell line resistant to TRAIL induced apoptosis and sensitive to TRAIL mediated proliferation (Baader et al., 2005), was tested (see Figure 13). In a first step, flow cytometric analysis confirmed that 91% ($M_2 - M_1$) of KELLY cells were successfully transfected with TRAIL targeting siRNA t_2. In a second step, cell growth analysis of transfected cells using CellScreen showed no difference in cell growth in the initial 24h. At 48h, however, control transfected cells measured cell densities of 18.000 cells per cm^2, while KELLY cells transfected with TRAIL targeting siRNA measured 8.000 cells per cm^2. A significant difference in cell density between KELLY cells transfected with TRAIL targeting siRNA t_2 and control siRNA transfected cells was confirmed by statistical analysis.

Taken together, growth behavior of transfected HEK, SHEP and KELLY cells differed in the course of the observation as demonstrated by the results of the present study. HEK and SHEP cells which were successfully transfected with TRAIL targeting siRNA t_2 showed growth behavior similar to control cells. The neuroblastoma cell line KELLY, however, demonstrated a significant difference in cell growth upon transfection with TRAIL targeting siRNA t_2. Compared to control cells KELLY cells which were transfected with siRNA t_2 showed a significantly decreased cell growth at 48h of growth analysis.

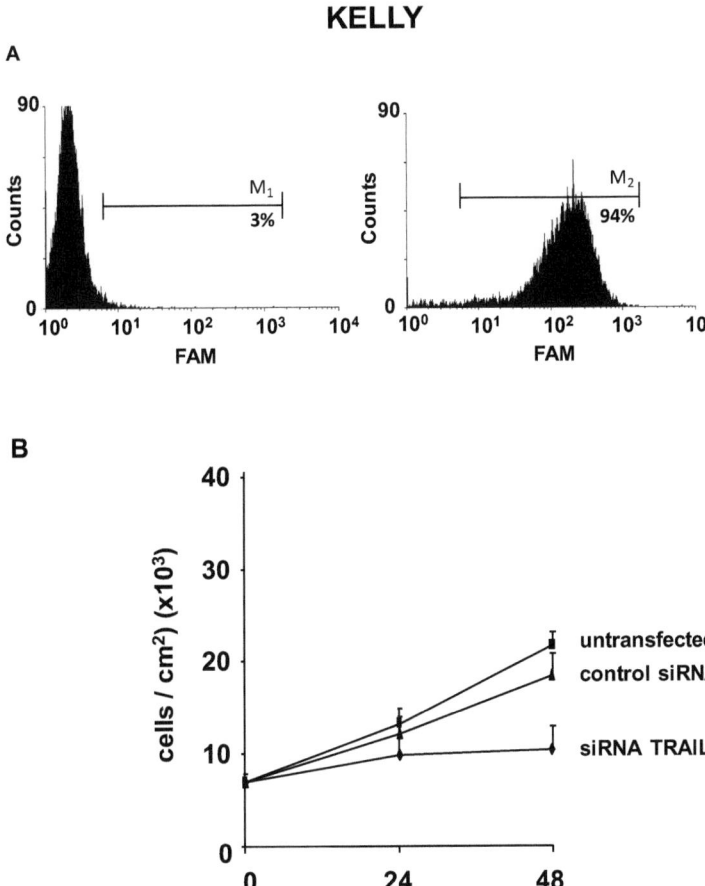

Figure 13. Transfection with TRAIL targeting siRNA shows an effect on cell growth in KELLY cells.
A. KELLY cells were treated for 48h with FAM labeled siRNA TRAIL and subjected to flow cytometric analysis. Histograms of a representative sample are illustrated. M_2 shows the fraction of transfected cells. B. KELLY cells were transfected for 48h with TRAIL targeting siRNA (siRNA TRAIL) and control siRNA and subjected to CellScreen measurement for 48h. Untransfected cells served as control. Error bars represent standard deviation of two independent experiments.

Results

6.4 KELLY cells and the effects of downregulation of endogenous TRAIL

To further characterize the proposed function of endogenous TRAIL for tumor cell growth, KELLY cells, which were transfected with TRAIL targeting siRNA, were further analyzed microscopically and flow cytometrically.

6.4.1 Reduction of cell growth

KELLY cells transfected with siRNA t_2 showed reduced cell growth compared to control cells, suggesting a function of endogenous TRAIL for tumor cell growth. To further analyze the described cell growth behavior and provide evidence that reduced cell growth was a result of endogenous TRAIL downregulation, I extended observation times and replicated the experiment using another TRAIL targeting siRNA. A direct verification of endogenous TRAIL downregulation on mRNA and protein level on KELLY cells, as performed in previous experiments of the present work (chapter 6.2.3), was technically not feasible due to very low expression levels of endogenous TRAIL in KELLY cells (see Figure 7). To exclude that the described cell growth behavior was a result of a sequence specific off-target effect of the interfering RNA (Jackson *et al.*, 2006), the experiment was reproduced using a TRAIL targeting siRNA of an alternative sequence.

To analyze growth behavior in more detail the exposure time of transfection medium and TRAIL targeting siRNA was prolonged to another 48h, and the observation time was extended to a total of 96h. Figure 14 illustrates the results of the extended cell growth analysis of KELLY cells transfected with TRAIL targeting siRNA t_2.

Results

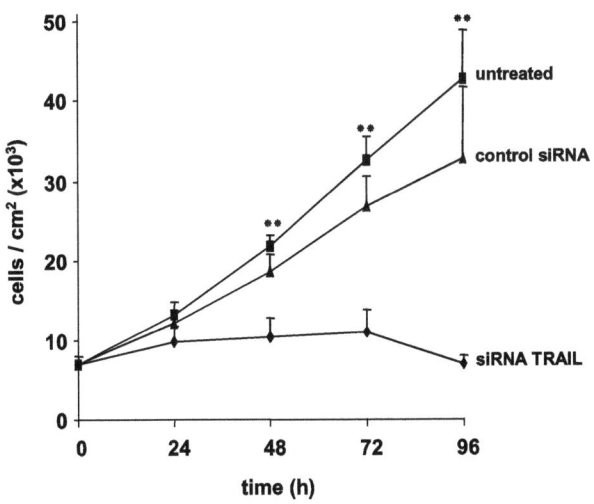

Figure 14. Decreased cell growth in KELLY cells transfected with TRAIL targeting siRNA.
KELLY cells were transfected with control siRNA or TRAIL targeting siRNA (siRNA TRAIL) at 0h and 48h. Cell growth was evaluated using CellScreen for 96h. Error bars represent standard deviation of three independent experiments. ** $P < 0.01$ (one-way RM ANOVA).

The results of the present study confirmed persistent cell growth reduction in KELLY cells transfected with TRAIL targeting siRNA t_2 at 72h and 96h (siRNA TRAIL). Significant differences of cell growth behavior of control transfected cells (control siRNA) and cells transfected with TRAIL targeting siRNA were detected at 48, 72 and 96h, indicating a stable manifestation. Cell densities of KELLY cells transfected with TRAIL targeting siRNA persisted at an equal level until 72h of transfection. At 96h a regressive growth behavior of KELLY cells was noticed, suggesting the occurrence of cell death.

In a next step, I repeated the experiment applying the TRAIL targeting siRNA t_1, which has been shown to have the second highest potential of reducing endogenous TRAIL on RNA level (chapter 6.2.3.1). Similar to the previous experiment KELLY cells were transfected at 0h and retransfected at 48h and thereafter subjected to cell growth measurement using CellScreen. Figure 15 illustrates results of the growth analysis of KELLY cells which were transfected with TRAIL targeting siRNA t_1.

Results

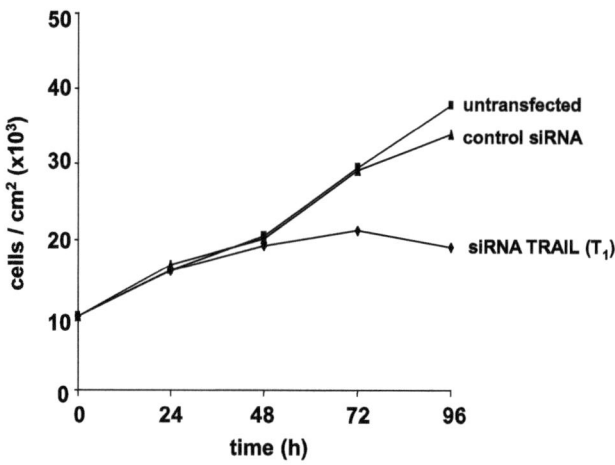

Figure 15. Decreased cell growth in KELLY cells transfected with a TRAIL targeting siRNA of a different sequence.
KELLY cells were transfected with control siRNA and a TRAIL targeting siRNA of a different sequence (siRNA TRAIL t_1) at 0h and 48h. Cell growth was evaluated for 96h using CellScreen. Shown is a representative of two independent experiments.

Cell growth analysis of KELLY cells which were transfected with an alternative TRAIL targeting siRNA (siRNA TRAIL t_1) revealed a similar reduction of cell density. Yet start of decreased cell growth was detected at 72h of observation, a later time point when compared to initial studies with KELLY cells transfected with TRAIL targeting siRNA t_2. Regressive cell growth was noted at 96h. The observation of a delayed decrease of cell growth, in comparison with the growth analysis of KELLY cells transfected with siRNA t_2, was compatible with the previously described reduced inhibiting potential of TRAIL targeting siRNA t_1 (see Figure 9).

Results

Taken together, the results of the present study show that the decrease in cellular density, which was seen in KELLY cells transfected with TRAIL targeting siRNA is stable over time and reproducible. Different TRAIL targeting siRNAs induced similar growth patterns in transfected KELLY cells. Previous experiments of the present work confirmed the potential of TRAIL targeting siRNA t_2 to downregulate endogenous TRAIL on mRNA and protein level independent of cell line used (6.2.3). In reference to these experiments I interpreted altered growth behavior of transfected KELLY cells, not to be a result of a sequence specific off-target effect of the siRNA used, but to be a direct effect of endogenous TRAIL downregulation. Furthermore, the extended analysis of cell growth of transfected KELLY cells yielded a regressive cell growth behavior at 96h, an observation which was suggestive of cell death.

6.4.2 Cell growth reduction is a result of cell death induction

After verifying the reproducibility and stability of the observed decrease of cell growth in KELLY cells upon the downregulation of endogenous TRAIL, I proceeded to investigate whether decreased cell numbers were a result of decreased cell growth or, alternatively, a result of an increase in cell death, which was suggested by a regressive growth behavior of KELLY cells, seen in previous studies of the present work (see Figure 14 and Figure 15).

To further characterize the observed cell growth behavior, KELLY cells were microscopically examined at 96h for morphological changes characteristic of cell death, such as cell shrinkage and membrane blebbing (Hengartner, 2000). Figure 16 illustrates microscopic evaluation of KELLY cells with and without the downregulation of endogenous TRAIL at 96h of cell growth analysis.

Results

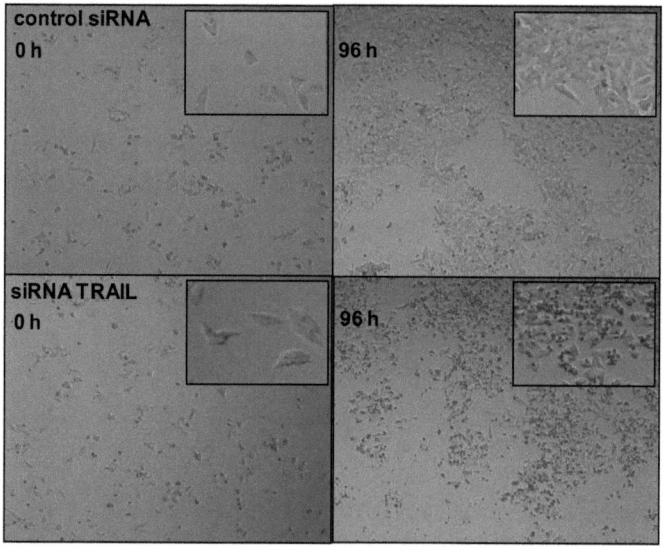

Figure 16. Reduced cell vitality in KELLY cells transfected with TRAIL targeting siRNA.
KELLY cells were transfected with control siRNA or TRAIL targeting siRNA (siRNA TRAIL) at 0h and 48h. Pictures of KELLY cells were taken at 0h (time of transfection) and at 96h in culture. Pictures of the upper panel show KELLY cells transfected with control siRNA. Pictures of the lower panel show KELLY cells transfected with TRAIL targeting siRNA (siRNA TRAIL).

At 96h of cell growth analysis KELLY cells transfected with TRAIL targeting siRNA showed a decrease in cell vitality when compared to cells transfected with non-silencing control siRNA. In-detail analysis by higher magnification revealed a rounded phenotype of Kelly cells with downregulated levels of endogenous TRAIL, suggesting the presence morphological changes specific of cell death (Wiley et al., 1980; Hengartner, 2000).

To confirm that the described changes were a manifestation of cell death, cells were subjected to a flow cytometric analysis to assess nuclear DNA fragmentation. DNA fragmentation is a process during apoptosis, in which nuclear DNA is cut into pieces and packaged away. Visualization of DNA fragmentation by flow cytometry was described as a reliable method for detecting cell death in past studies (Nicoletti et al., 1991; Darzynkiewicz et al., 1992). Figure 17 illustrates the result of the present experiment.

Results

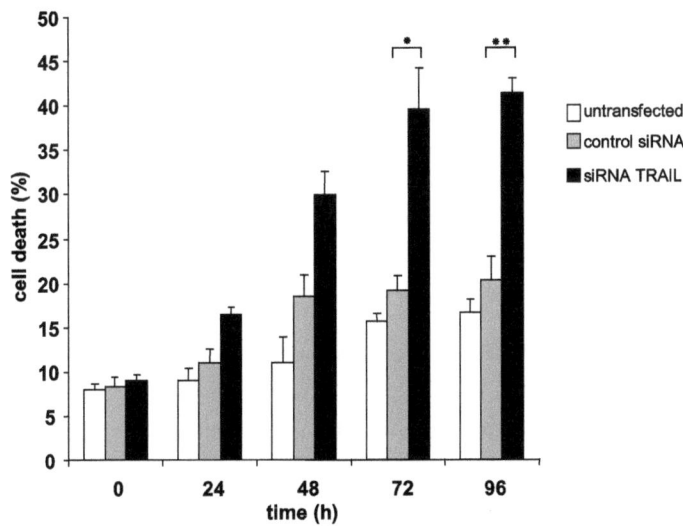

Figure 17. Increase in cell death in KELLY cells transfected with TRAIL targeting siRNA.
KELLY cells were transfected with TRAIL targeting siRNA (siRNA TRAIL) or control siRNA at 0h and 48h. Untreated KELLY cells served as control. At 0h, 24, 48, 72 and 96h after transfection cells were treated with Nicoletti buffer and subjected to cell death analysis using flow cytometry. Columns represent percentage of cell death of respective cell sample. Error bars represent standard deviation of three independent experiments. *$P < 0.05$, **$P < 0.01$ (one-way RM ANOVA).

Flow cytometric analysis performed at the time of transfection (0h) and at 24h, 48h, 72h and 96h after transfection yielded significant differences in the occurrence of cell death between KELLY cells transfected with TRAIL targeting siRNA (siRNA TRAIL) and control transfected cells (control siRNA). At the start of transfection both transfected and non-transfected KELLY cells showed similar cell death rates. However, at 72h and 96h after transfection cell death rates significantly increased in a time dependant manner in KELLY cells transfected with TRAIL targeting siRNA (siRNA TRAIL). 40 % of KELLY cells subjected to the transient downregulation of endogenous TRAIL showed cell death specific morphological changes at 96h in comparison to 20% of control transfected cells. Cell death rates of untreated KELLY cells accounted for 15% of cell death rates at 96h.

Results

Taken together, the results of the present study showed that the downregulation of endogenous TRAIL by means of RNA interference induced morphological changes in Kelly cells which were consistent with morphological changes seen in cell death. This observation was confirmed by a flow cytometric analysis, showing an increase in nuclear DNA fragmentation, a reliable marker of cell death, in KELLY cells transfected with TRAIL targeting siRNA. The data of the present study suggested that the previously observed reduction of cell growth in KELLY cells, subjected to the downregulation of endogenous TRAIL, was a result of the induction of cell death.

6.4.3 Soluble TRAIL rescues cell death induced by the downregulation of endogenous TRAIL

The experiments of the present work showed that the downregulation of endogenous TRAIL induced cell death in the neuroblastoma cell line KELLY and lead therefore to a decrease in tumor growth. In the following study I investigated the potential of soluble TRAIL to replace the function of endogenous TRAIL and prevent cell death induced by the downregulation of endogenous TRAIL. For this purpose levels of endogenous TRAIL were once more reduced by transfecting KELLY cells with TRAIL targeting siRNA (t_{siRNA}) for 48h. For the following 24h I treated KELLY cells with 10 ng/ml of soluble TRAIL, a concentration, which was shown to induce cell growth in KELLY cells in previous experiments of this study (chapter 6.1). Flow cytometric analysis followed 24h after completing transfection at a total observation time of 72h. Figure 18 illustrates the results of the experiment.

Results

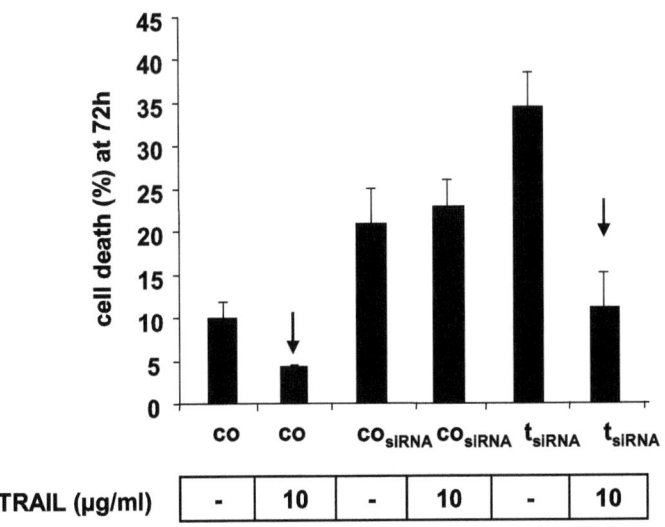

Figure 18. Treatment with soluble TRAIL rescues KELLY cells which were transfected with TRAIL targeting siRNA.
Kelly cells were transfected with control siRNA (co_{siRNA}) or TRAIL targeting siRNA (t_{siRNA}) for 48h. Thereafter cells were stimulated with 10 ng/ml TRAIL (10) or left unstimulated (-) for the following 24h. Cells were treated with Nicoletti buffer subsequently and subjected to flow cytometric analysis to evaluate cell death. Untransfected KELLY cells served as control. Columns represent percentage of cell death. Error bars represent standard deviation of three independent experiments.

Flow cytometric analysis of nuclear DNA fragmentation in KELLY cells treated with TRAIL confirmed the previously described pro-survival function of soluble TRAIL by showing a reduction of cell death in non-transfected TRAIL treated cells. Furthermore, KELLY cells subjected to the transfection with TRAIL targeting siRNA and subsequent TRAIL treatment (t_{siRNA}) showed decreased occurrence rates of cell death measured by flow cytometry. The occurrence of cell death in these cells decreased to levels which were comparable to untreated control cells (co). Cell death rates decreased to lower levels than rates of control transfected cells, indicating that soluble TRAIL prevented apoptotic cell death induced by endogenous TRAIL down regulation and in addition exerted a further pro-survival/ pro-proliferative function on KELLY cells. Control transfected KELLY cells (c_{siRNA}) did not show a significant difference in cell death occurrence in TRAIL treated and non-treated samples. This

Results

observation suggested the presence of cell death, which was unresponsive to TRAIL treatment.

Taken together the data of the present study confirmed that soluble TRAIL, which has been shown to have a pro-survival function in previous studies, rescued KELLY cells with downregulated levels of endogenous TRAIL and by this means successfully replaced the putative survival promoting function of endogenous TRAIL in KELLY cells.

6.4.4 Cell death is mediated by caspases

Morphological changes and DNA fragmentation occurring after the downregulation of endogenous TRAIL were features suggesting cell death in the neuroblastoma cell line KELLY. Cell death is executed either in a programmed manner, as for instance in form of apoptosis, or in a non-programmed manner, as for instance in form of necrosis. Characteristic features of the programmed cell death apoptosis are, next to morphologic changes, the activation of caspases (Degterev et al., 2003).

In the following experiment cell death induced by the downregulation of endogenous TRAIL was analyzed in more detail. Caspase activation was measured to assess for apoptotic cell death. If Kelly cells died by apoptosis upon downregulation of endogenous TRAIL, and caspases, as the central mediators of apoptosis, are inhibited, then downregulation of endogenous TRAIL should have no effect on KELLY cells. To investigate this hypothesis I subjecting KELLY cells to treatment with the pancaspase inhibitor Q-VD prior to the downregulation of endogenous TRAIL by means of interfering RNA and subjected cells to flow cytometric analysis of cell death. The pancaspase inhibitor Q-VD irreversibly binds and inactivates downstream caspases 1, 3, 8 and 9 (Caserta et al., 2003). Figure 19 illustrates the results of the flow cytometric analysis.

Results

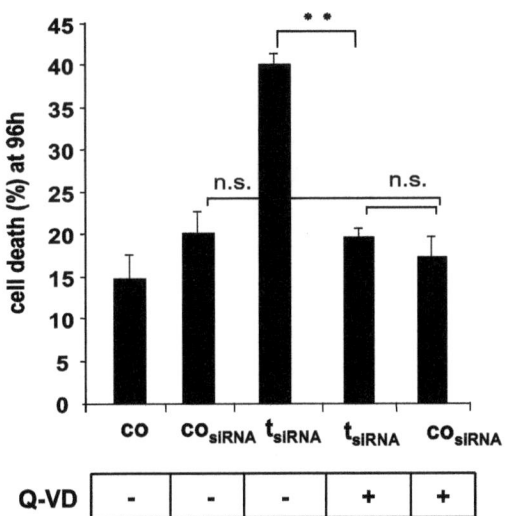

Figure 19. The Pancaspase inhibitor Q-VD prevents cell death of KELLY cells induced by the transfection of TRAIL targeting siRNA.
KELLY cells were transfected with control siRNA (co_{siRNA}) and Trail targeting siRNA (t_{siRNA}) at 0h and 48h. Q-VD was added to KELLY cells 1 h prior to transfection and at 48h to reach a concentration of 50µM. Cells were subjected to cell death analysis using flow cytometry at 96h. Untransfected cells served as controls (co). Columns represent the percentage of cell death which was measured at 96h. Error bars show the standard deviation of three independent experiments. **$P < 0.01$(one-way RM ANOVA). n.s.= not significant.

In accordance to data of previous experiments (Figure 17) flow cytometric analysis of cell death at 96h after transfection yielded cell death rates of 42% in KELLY cells, which were transfected with TRAIL targeting siRNA (t_{siRNA}). As expected cell death rates were significantly higher when compared to cell death rates of control transfected cells. Further analysis demonstrated that the pre-treatment of KELLY cells with pancaspase inhibitor prevented an increase in cell death upon downregulation of endogenous TRAIL. Pretreated KELLY cells had similar cell death rates as control transfected cells. No significant difference in cell death was detected in control transfected cells with or without prior caspase inhibition.

Results

Taken together, as control transfected KELLY cells and KELLY cells transfected with TRAIL targeting siRNA showed similar rates of cell death upon treatment with pancaspase inhibitor Q-VD, the results of the present study demonstrated that pancaspase inhibitor successfully prevented cell death induced by the downregulation of endogenous TRAIL. No significant differences in cell death occurred in control transfected cells with or without prior caspase inhibition, showing that caspase activation was not involved in spontaneously occurring cell death of KELLY cells. As caspases are key mediators of the programmed cell death apoptosis (Hengartner, 2000), caspase activation in KELLY cells suggested the induction of apoptosis by the downregulation of endogenous TRAIL. This data therefore suggested an anti-apoptotic function of endogenous TRAIL.

In summary, microscopic and flow cytometric analysis provided evidence that the initially observed decrease of cell growth in the neuroblastoma cell line KELLY, subjected to the downregulation of endogenous TRAIL, was a result of cell death induction. Cell death induced by the downregulation of endogenous TRAIL was successfully rescued by soluble TRAIL and dependent on caspase activation. Taken together, the data of the present work provided first evidence for a putative role of endogenous TRAIL as a pro-survival /anti-apoptotic factor in the neuroblastoma cell line KELLY, a human cancer cell line resistant to TRAIL induced apoptosis.

Discussion

7 Discussion

The pro-proliferative and pro-survival effect of soluble TRAIL has been described as a new adverse effect of TRAIL therapy in past studies (Ehrhardt *et al.*, 2003). A positive correlation between endogenous TRAIL expression and cancer cell growth, in terms of decreased disease-specific survival, has been shown in renal cell carcinoma, a cancer cell line resistant to TRAIL induced apoptosis (Oya et al., 2001; Macher-Goeppinger *et al.*, 2009). The present data provided first evidence for the function of endogenous TRAIL as an endogenous pro-survival factor of the neuroblastoma cell line KELLY, a human cell line resistant to TRAIL induced apoptosis. By means of cell death analysis endogenous TRAIL downregulation has been shown to result in an increase of cell death in the neuroblastoma cell line KELLY. The present data thus suggested that endogenous TRAIL expression is an important intrinsic stimulus for the cell survival and cell growth of KELLY cells. This novel, up-to-date unknown function of endogenous TRAIL is of great importance for the understanding of the role of endogenous TRAIL in tumor cell survival and for its potential as a novel target in cancer therapy.

7.1 Substantial effect of the down regulation of TRAIL on cell viability

Downregulation of endogenous TRAIL resulted in an impressive cell growth decrease in KELLY cells as measured using the automated microscope CellScreen. This was an unexpected observation, as previous studies of our research laboratory and initial studies of the present work showed that TRAIL had a significant, yet small proliferation inducing effect on KELLY cells. With the down regulation of endogenous TRAIL our research group anticipated a cell growth decrease of similar extent. Yet CellScreen data showed that the downregulation of endogenous TRAIL had a deleterious effect on KELLY cells. The seemingly disproportional effect of endogenous TRAIL and soluble TRAIL on KELLY cells measured by CellScreen initiated further in-detail studies. Flow cytometric analysis, measuring cell death, proved that the downregulation of endogenous TRAIL induced cell death and lead to decreased cell survival. Furthermore, by this means an equally strong effect of soluble TRAIL and endogenous TRAIL was shown, as soluble TRAIL fully rescued cell death induced by the downregulation of endogenous TRAIL. Taken together, we concluded that the use of CellScreen is a valuable approach to study cell proliferation in

Discussion

culture, but the present data suggested that it is an unreliable tool to measure cell viability and survival.

7.2 Cell-type specificity of the function of endogenous TRAIL

The downregulation of endogenous TRAIL was carried out by transient transfection of TRAIL targeting interfering RNA. By this means the production of endogenous TRAIL was identified as a critical factor for cell survival, but the experiments of the present work showed that this observation was limited to the human neuroblastoma cell line KELLY.

Different reasons can account for this limited detection. The limited occurrence of the pro-survival function of endogenous TRAIL on KELLY cells, but not on two additional human cancer cell lines, may have been a result of an imprecise detection of a generally occurring function of endogenous TRAIL. Initial optimization studies of the present work proved the potential of the applied siRNA to lower endogenous TRAIL on mRNA and protein level. Screening different cell lines showed that KELLY cells naturally produce very little amounts of endogenous TRAIL. Subjecting KELLY cells to transient transfection with RNA interference possibly lead to exceptionally low levels of endogenous TRAIL. It can be assumed that only a complete downregulation of endogenous TRAIL sufficiently evoked an apoptotic cell death response. As other human cancer cell lines showed naturally high levels of endogenous TRAIL, the present studies presumably never lead to a comparable level of downregulation of endogenous TRAIL in the cell lines tested. Therefore the methodology applied in this work may have been ineffective to induce equally low levels of endogenous TRAIL among the human cancer cell lines and the occurrence of the pro-survival function of endogenous TRAIL may have been underestimated.

Discussion

It is also possible that the significance of endogenous TRAIL for cell survival is a cell-type specific phenomenon of cells which show TRAIL-induced proliferation such as KELLY cells. Cell-type specific functions of proteins are a common observation. Furthermore cellular heterogeneity has been shown in the neuroblastoma cell lines (Ross and Spengler, 2004). The present findings therefore may describe a function of endogenous TRAIL which due to cellular heterogeneity is only applicable to the neuroblastoma cell line KELLY.

Apart from that, a group-specific function of endogenous TRAIL is conceivable. The pro-survival function of endogenous TRAIL may be limited to cancers which show TRAIL mediated proliferation, among them the neuroblastoma cell line KELLY. As past studies showed that selected cancer cells (SHEP, HEK) are not sensitive to TRAIL mediated proliferation (Ehrhardt *et al*, 2003), the present work proved that the downregulation of endogenous TRAIL had no effect on their cell growth. According to this data the significance of endogenous TRAIL for tumor cell survival may be a group-specific phenomenon.

7.3 Role of endogenous TRAIL for cancer cells

The pro-proliferative function of soluble TRAIL has been widely recognized. In the present work, the role of endogenous, membrane-bound, TRAIL for tumor cell growth and cell survival was investigated. Results of the present work showed that reduced expression of endogenous TRAIL lead to a cell death response in the neuroblastoma cell line KELLY, which in turn was rescued by treatment with soluble TRAIL. Therefore, it is presumed that the expression of endogenous TRAIL is necessary for the survival of KELLY cells.

In the past, the role of endogenous TRAIL in tumor biology has been suggested. Clinical studies had shown that increased TRAIL expression in renal-cell carcinoma is associated with decreased disease-specific survival (Macher-Goeppinger *et al.*, 2009). Furthermore, studies observed that the expression of endogenous TRAIL is associated with an aggressive and proliferative phenotype in human melanoma cells (Bron *et al.*, 2004). This data suggested an association between endogenous TRAIL expression and tumor burden, or tumor cell growth. The data of the present study provide first evidence of a direct effect of endogenous TRAIL on tumor cell growth. Down regulated TRAIL expression lead to a significant decrease of cell growth by increasing apoptotic cell death in the human neuroblastoma cell line, KELLY. TRAIL treatment, in turn, rescued cell death induced by the down regulation of endogenous TRAIL. With this data the present work provided first evidence that the expression of endogenous TRAIL was essential for the viability of the selected human cancer cell line

Discussion

KELLY and suggested an important role of endogenous TRAIL for the cell survival of cancers resistant to TRAIL-induced apoptosis. Further studies under N. Ishimura complement the present data, showing that endogenous TRAIL is up regulated in cholangiocarcinoma cells, which show increased cell migration and invasion upon TRAIL treatment (Ishimura et al., 2006).

7.4 Pro-survival function of several members of the TNF-family

Next to the proliferation-inducing effect of soluble TRAIL further members of the TNF/TNFR-superfamily have been acknowledged to exert a pro-proliferative function on cancer and non-cancerous cells (Vinay and Kwon, 2009). In-vitro studies showed that the member of the TNF/TNFR-superfamily, Tumor necrosis factor-α (TNF-α), induces proliferation on cancer cell lines derived from osteosarcoma and leukemia (Kirstein et al., 1988; Ferrajoli et al., 2002). Investigations around C. Tselepis emphasized the role of TNF-α as an autocrine and paracrine growth factor of Barett's adenocarcinoma. C. Tselepis showed that a direct effect of TNF-α stimulation on the intracellular c-myc expression of esophageal cells exists, linking the activation of c-myc to the observed pro-proliferative effect of TNF-α (Tselepis et al., 2002). In further investigations B.C. Bernhart identified CD95, also a member of the TNF/TNFR-superfamily, to exert a pro-tumorigenic effect on apoptosis resistant cancers, by increasing cancer cell motility and invasiveness. The tumor enhancing effect of CD95 was described as a result of the stimulation of membrane-bound CD95 by several ligands (Bernhart et al., 2004).

Furthermore, several members of the TNF/TNFR-superfamily have been shown to exert an intrinsic pro-survival function on cell growth and cell survival. For instance, investigations under H.J. Gruss and S.K. Dower showed that members of the TNF/TNFR-superfamily, CD40 and CD 40 Ligand (CD40L), have a pro-survival function on immune cells. CD40 and CD40L are membrane-bound proteins which are expressed on the surface of B- and T-lymphocytes. The interaction of CD40 with CD40L activates immune cells and leads to their proliferation and protection against apoptosis. Defect or absence of CD40 or CD40L results in the disruption of protein interaction, the induction of cell death and thus the development of an immunodeficient state (Gruss and Dower, 1995; Baker and Reddy, 1996). Furthermore, Ox-40, also a member of the TNF/TNFR-superfamily, has been recognized as an essential factor for long-term survival of T-lymphocytes. In-vitro studies showed that the knockdown of OX-40

Discussion

in activated CD-4+ T-lymphocytes lead to the loss of anti-apoptotic factor Bcl-2 and therefore to the induction of apoptosis within 4-8 days (Rogers et al., 2001). The data of the present work further showed that the downregulation of endogenous TRAIL lead to the induction of apoptotic cell death in the neuroblastoma cell line KELLY. With this data a putative function of endogenous TRAIL, a member of the TNF/TNFR-superfamily, as an intrinsic pro-survival factor was suggested.

7.5 Mechanisms of the pro-survival function of TNF-family members

The pro-survival and pro-cancerogenic effect of TNF-α, CD95 ligands and TRAIL has been described to be mediated through direct stimulation of the aforementioned ligands with its receptors. With the data of the presenting work, we provided evidence that endogenous TRAIL exerts an intrinsic pro-survival function on selected cells.

So far, it remains unknown how endogenous TRAIL expression protects the neuroblastoma cell line from apoptotic cell death. Different pro-survival mechanisms of the TNF/TNFR-superfamily members have been well-recognized. In reference to the TNF/TNFR-superfamily members CD40 and CD40L, it is conceivable that endogenous TRAIL expression leads to a reciprocal interaction of TRAIL with its receptor, activating intracellular pro-survival factors in a paracrine manner. Furthermore, the intracellular interaction of endogenous TRAIL with its receptor may bestow endogenous TRAIL the function as an intrinsic survival factor. The intracellular expression of TRAIL receptors on organelles, such as the Golgi apparatus, has been described in past studies (Zhang et al., 2000). Further mechanisms have been well recognized for the TNF/TNFR-superfamily member OX-40. The activation of OX-40, a membrane-bound surface receptor, has been shown to induce the expression of BCL-2, a well known anti-apoptotic factor and by this means contribute to the survival of T-cells (Rogers et al., 2011). Comparable interactions have been described in past studies for endogenous TRAIL, showing that the expression of endogenous TRAIL is linked to NF-κB activation on t-lymphocytes (Baetu et al., 2001).

Discussion

7.6 Future perspective

TRAIL has been identified as a promising anti-cancer drug in the past (Walzak et al., 1999; Ashkenazi et al., 1999). But rising resistance to TRAIL therapy has initiated a growing demand for additional therapeutic approaches. The present work provides first evidence for the potential of endogenous TRAIL as a novel therapeutic target of cancer therapy. Yet to evaluate the potential role of endogenous TRAIL for cellular growth and survival, current investigations need to integrate further models of cancer. Stable transfection of endogenous TRAIL targeting interfering RNA and those targeting potential interaction partners, would allow a further molecular characterization of the apoptotic effect induced by downregulation of endogenous TRAIL on different cancer entities. In addition, investigations on primary cells would be of special interest, to allow the acquisition and analysis of larger datasets and by this means reliably assess the frequency of occurrence.

7.7 Potential relevance as a novel approach of cancer therapy

The efficiency of loco-regional siRNA treatment of different cancer entities have been shown in different in-vitro and in-vivo cancer models (Tong et al., 2005; Hosaka et al., 2006; Morales et al., 2007). Systemic application of siRNA for cancer therapy is an emerging therapeutic tool and currently synthetic siRNAs are being evaluated in clinical Phase1 trials (Davis et al., 2010). The data of the present work provided new evidence for the potential of the downregulation of endogenous TRAIL by TRAIL targeting siRNAs (siRNAs) as an additional therapeutic approach in cancer therapy directed against cancers resistant to TRAIL-induced apoptosis. The data of the present work showed that small interfering RNAs targeting endogenous TRAIL induce an apoptotic cell death response in the neuroblastoma cell line KELLY and by this means effectively reduced the number of cancer cells. This up-to-date unknown effect of the downregulation of endogenous TRAIL on cancer cells is of great importance for the understanding of the role of endogenous TRAIL in tumor biology and for its potential as a novel therapeutic target in cancer therapy. In the light of the emerging clinical applicability of siRNAs in cancer therapy, the apoptotic function of TRAIL targeting siRNAs on selected cancer cells provides an interesting therapeutic approach for patient with cancers resistant to TRAIL-induced apoptosis and high expression of endogenous TRAIL.

Summary

8 Summary

Tumor necrosis factor-related apoptosis-inducing ligand (TRAIL) has been shown to exert an unexpected pro-survival, pro-proliferative and pro-invasive effect on a subset of human cancer cell lines. Recent clinical studies report that increased expression of endogenous TRAIL is associated with decreased disease-specific survival in renal cell carcinoma and cholangiocarcinoma which are resistant to TRAIL induced apoptosis. The present work investigated the role of endogenous TRAIL as an intrinsic growth factor in apoptosis-resistant human cancer cells.

Several cell lines derived from solid human tumors were studied, among them the neuroblastoma cell line KELLY, a cancer cell line resistant to TRAIL-induced apoptosis. First, to investigate whether TRAIL-knockdown could inhibit cell growth, the use of small interfering RNAs (siRNA) for endogenous TRAIL was established and a successful knockdown was verified on both mRNA and protein level. Second, the functional impact of the knockdown of endogenous TRAIL was investigated by measuring cell growth and cell death after transfection: Interestingly, the human neuroblastoma cell line KELLY unexpectedly showed markedly reduced cell growth upon knockdown of endogenous TRAIL. Furthermore, knockdown of TRAIL induced cell death in KELLY cells, which was dependent on caspase-signaling and rescued by the addition of soluble TRAIL. Thus, endogenous TRAIL functions as an intrinsic survival and growth factor in the neuroblastoma cell line KELLY. The present work provided first evidence that the expression of endogenous TRAIL can be specifically downregulated through siRNA knockdown to inhibit survival and growth of cancer cells in-vitro, which are resistant to TRAIL induced apoptosis.

The present data strongly supports the potential of endogenous TRAIL to function as a novel therapeutic target in cancer therapy. In the light of the emerging clinical use of siRNAs for cancer therapy, targeting TRAIL by RNA interference may provide a valuable treatment approach for patients with cancers resistant to TRAIL induced apoptosis and high expression levels of endogenous TRAIL.

9 Zusammenfassung

Tumor necrosis factor related apoptosis-inducing ligand (TRAIL) zeigt eine unerwartete Wachstums-, Überlebens- und Invasionsfördernde Wirkung auf einzelne Apoptose-resistente humane Tumorzelllinien. Gleichzeitig wurde in klinischen Studien belegt, dass der Nachweis einer gesteigerten Expression von endogenem TRAIL im Tumorgewebe von Patienten mit Nierenzellkarzinomen und Cholangiokarzinomen mit einer Verminderung der tumorspezifischen Überlebensrate vergesellschaftet ist. In der vorliegenden Arbeit wurde die Bedeutung von endogenen TRAIL als intrinsischer Wachstumsfaktor auf Apoptose-resistente Tumorzellen untersucht.

Die Analyse umfasste Zelllinien solider Tumoren, insbesondere die humane Neuroblastoma Zelllinie KELLY, die eine Resistenz gegenüber TRAIL-induzierter Apoptose aufweist. In einem ersten Schritt wurde ein effizienter TRAIL-knockdown mittels *small interfering RNAs* (siRNA) methodologisch etabliert und die erfolgreiche Abregulierung von endogenen TRAIL auf mRNA- und Proteinebene nachgewiesen. In einem zweiten Schritt wurde die funktionelle Auswirkung der Abregulation von endogenen TRAIL auf das Proliferations- und Apoptoseverhalten der Tumorzellen untersucht: Interessanterweise führte der spezifische knockdown von TRAIL mittels siRNA zu einer unmittelbaren Proliferationshemmung der Neuroblastoma Zelllinie KELLY. Darüber hinaus wurde durch den knockdown von endogenem TRAIL ein Caspase-abhängiger Zelltod der KELLY Zellen induziert. Die Zugabe von exogenem TRAIL konnte die Apoptose der KELLY Zellen nach Behandlung mit TRAIL-siRNA effizient vermindern. Endogenes TRAIL wirkt somit als intrinsischer Überlebens- und Wachstumsfaktor für die Neuroblastoma Zelllinie KELLY. Die vorliegende Arbeit zeigt erstmals, dass die Expression von endogenem TRAIL durch die Anwendung von siRNA erfolgreich reduziert werden kann und das TRAIL-knockdown das Wachstum einer Apoptose-resistenten Zelllinie inhibiert.

Diese Ergebnisse unterstützen die Hypothese, dass TRAIL einen potentiellen Angriffspunkt für die Behandlung Apoptose-resistenter Tumoren darstellen könnte. Vor dem Hintergrund der beginnenden klinischen Anwendung von siRNA könnte RNA-Interferenz mit TRAIL einen interessanten Ansatzpunkt für die Behandlung von Tumoren mit einer Resistenz gegenüber TRAIL induzierter Apoptose sowie einer hoher Expression von endogenen TRAIL darstellen.

10 References

Abadie A and Wietzerbin J. Involvement of TNF-related apoptotis-inducing lingand (TRAIL) induction in interferon gamma-mediated apoptosis in Ewing tumor cells. *Ann N Y Acad Sci* 1010: 117-120. (2003).

Ahmad M and Shi Y. TRAIL-induced apoptosis of thyroid cancer cells: potential for therapeutic intervention. *Oncogene* 19: 3363-3371. (2000).

Alexopoulou L, Holt AC, Medzhitov R and Flavell RA. Recognition of double-stranded RNA and activation of NF-kappaB by Toll-like receptor 3. *Nature* 413, 732-738. (2001).

Ashkenazi A, Pai RC, Fong S, Leung S, Lawrence DA, Marsters SA, Blackie C, Chang L, McMurtrey AE, Herbert A, DeForge L, Koumenis IL, Lewis D, Harris L, Bussiere J, Koeppen H, Shahrokh Z and Schwall RH. Safety and antitumor activity of recombinant soluble Apo2ligand. *J Clin Invest* 104(2): 155-162. (1999).

Ashkenazi A. Targeting death and decoy receptors of the tumour-necrosis factor superfamily. *Nat Rev Cancer* 2(6): 420-430. (2002).

Baader E, Toloczko A, Fuchs U, Schmid I, Ehrhardt H, Debatin KM and Jeremias I. Tumor necrosis factor-related apoptosis-inducing ligand-mediated proliferation of tumor cells with receptor-proximal apoptosis defects. *Cancer Res* 65(17): 7888-7895. (2005).

Baetu TM, Kwon H, Sharma S, Grandvaux N and Hiscott J. Disruption of NF-kappaB signaling reveals a novel role for NF-kappaB in the regulation of TNF-related apoptosis-inducing ligand expression. *J Immunol* 167 (6): 3164-3173. (2001).

Baker SJ, Reddy EP. Transducers of life and death: TNF receptor superfamily and associated proteins. *Oncogene* 12(1):1-9. (1996).

Belka C, Schmid B, Marini P, Durand E, Rudner J, Faltin H, Bamberg M, Schulze-Osthoff K and Budach W. Sensitization of resistant lymphoma cells to irradiation-induced apoptosis by the death ligand TRAIL. *Oncogene* 20 (17): 2190-2196. (2001).

Belyanskaya LL, Ziogas A, Hopkins-Donaldson S, Kurtz S, Simon HU, Stahel R and Zangemeister-Wittke U. Trail-induced survival and proliferation of SCLC cells is mediated by ERK and dependent on TRAIL-R2/DR5 expression in the absence of caspase-8. *Lung Cancer* 60(3): 355-365. (2008).

Besch R, Poeck H, Hohenauer T, Senft D, Hacker G, Berking C, Hornung V, Endres S, Ruzicka T, Rothenfusser S and Hartmann G. Proapoptotic signaling induced by RIG-I and MDA-5 results in type 1 interferon-independent apoptosis in human melanoma cells. *J Clin Invest* 119(8): 2399-2411. (2009).

Bretz JD, Rymaszewski M, Arscott PL, Myc A, Ain KB, Thompson NW and Baker JR, Jr. TRAIL death pathway expression and induction in thyroid follicular cells. *J Biol Chem* 274(33): 23627-23632. (1999).

Bron LP, Scolyer RA, Thompson JF, Hersey P. Histological expression of tumour necrosis factor-related apoptosis-inducing ligand (TRAIL) in human primary melanoma. *Pathology* 36(6):561-5. (2004).

Caponigro F, Basile M, de R, V and Normanno N. New drugs in cancer therapy, National Tumor Institute, Naples, 17-18 June 2004. *Anticancer Drugs* 16(2): 211-221. (2005).

References

Caserta, T. M., A. N. Smith, A. D. Gultice, M. A. Reedy, and T. L. Brown. Q-VD-OPh, a broad spectrum caspase inhibitor with potent antiapoptotic properties. *Apoptosis* 8:345-352. (2003).

Cho YS, Challa S, Clancy L and Chan FK. Lipopolysaccharide-induced expression of TRAIL promotes dendritic cell differentiation. *Immunology* 130(4): 504-515. (2010).

Chou AH, Tsai HF, Lin LL, Hsieh SL, Hsu PI and Hsu PN. Enhanced proliferation and increased IFN-gamma production in Tcells by signal transduced trhough TNF-related apoptosis-inducing ligand. *J Immunol* 167(3): 1347-1352. (2001).

Darzynkiewicz Z, Bruno S, Del BG, Gorczyca W, Hotz MA, Lassota P and Traganos F. Features of apoptotic cells measured by flow cytometry. *Cytometry* 13(8): 795-808. (1992).

Davis ME, Zuckerman JE, Choi CH, Seligson D, Tolcher A, Alabi CA, Yen Y, Heidel JD, Ribas A. Evidence of RNAi in humans from systemically administered siRNA via targeted nanoparticles. *Nature* 464(7291):1067-70. (2010).

Decaudin D, Marzo I, Brenner C and Kroemer G. Mitochondria in chemotherapy-induced apoptosis: a prospective novel target of cancer therapy (review). *Int J Oncol* 12(1): 141-152. (1998).

Degterev A, Boyce M and Yuan J. A decade of caspases. *Oncogene* 22(53): 8543-8567. (2003).

Dykxhoorn DM, Novina CD and Sharp PA. Killing the messenger: short RNAs that silence gene expression. *Nat Rev Mol Cell Biol* 4(6): 457-467. (2003).

Ehrhardt H, Fulda S, Schmid I, Hiscott J, Debatin KM and Jeremias I. TRAIL induced survival and proliferation in cancer cells resistant towards TRAIL-induced apoptosis mediated by NF-kappaB. *Oncogene* 22(25): 3842-3852. (2003).

Ehrlich S, Infante-Duarte C, Seeger B and Zipp F. Regulation of soluble and surface-bound TRAIL in human T cells, B cells, and monocytes. *Cytokine* 24(6): 244-253. (2003).

Elbashir SM, Harborth J, Lendeckel W, Yalcin A, Weber K and Tuschl T. Duplexes of 21-nucleotide RNAs mediate RNA interference in cultured mammalian cells. *Nature* 411(6836): 494-498. (2001).

Falschlehner C, Emmerich CH, Gerlach B and Walczak H. TRAIL signalling: decisions between life and death. *Int J Biochem Cell Biol* 39(7-8): 1462-1475. (2007).

Fanger NA, Maliszewski CR, Schooley K and Griffith TS. Human dendritic cells mediate cellular apoptosis via tumor necrosis factor-related apoptosis-inducing ligand (TRAIL). *J Exp Med* 190(8): 1155-1164. (1999).

Ferlay J, Shin HR, Bray F, Forman D, Mathers C and Parkin DM. Estimates of worldwide burden of cancer in 2008: GLOBOSCAN 2008. *Int J Cancer*. (2010).

Ferrajoli A, Keating MJ, Manshouri T, Giles FJ, Dey A, Estrov Z, Koller CA, Kurzrock R, Thomas DA, Faderl S, Lerner S, O'Brien S, Albitar M. The clinical significance of tumor necrosis factor-alpha plasma level in patients having chronic lymphocytic leukemia. *Blood* 100(4):1215-9. (2002).

Fulda S and Debatin KM. Targeting apoptosis pathways in cancer therapy. *Curr Cancer Drug Targets* 4: 569-576. (2004)

Fulda S and Debatin KM. Extrinsic versus intrinsic apoptosis pathways in anticancer chemotherapy. *Oncogene* 25(34): 4798-4811. (2006).

References

Fulda S, Küfer MU, Meyer E, Van Valen F, Dockhorn-Dworniczak B and Debatin KM. Sensitization for death receptor- or drug-induced apoptosis by re-expression of caspase-8 through demethylation or gene transfer. *Oncogene* 20(41): 5865-5877. (2001).

Ganten TM, Haas TL, Sykora J, Stahl H, Sprick MR, Fas SC, Krueger A, Weigand MA, Grosse-Wilde A, Stremmel W, Krammer PH and Walczak H. Enhanced caspase-8 recruitment to and activation at the DISC is critical for sensitization of human hepatocellular carcinoma cells to TRAIL-induced apoptosis by chemotherapeutic drugs. *Cell Death Differ* 11(Suppl1): 86-96. (2004).

Green DR and Kroemer G. The pathophysiology of mitochondrial cell death. *Science* 305(5684): 626-629. (2004).

Grosse-Wilde A and Kemp CJ. Matastasis suppressor function of tumor necrosis factor-related apoptosis-inducing ligand-R in mice: implications for TRAIL-based therapy in humans? *Cancer Res* 68(15): 6035-6037. (2008)

Gruss HJ and Dower SK. The TNF ligand superfamily and its relevance for human diseases. *Cytokines Mol Ther* 1(12): 75-105. (1995).

Halaas O, Liabakk NB, Vik R, Beninati C, Henneke P, Sundan A and Espevik T. Monocytes stimulated with group B streptococci and interferons release tumour necrosis factor-related apoptosis-inducing ligand. *Scand J Immunol* 60(1-2): 74-81. (2004).

Harada K, Sato Y, Itatsu K, Isse K, Ikeda H, Yasoshima M, Zen Y, Matsui A and Nakanuma Y. Innate immune response to double-stranded RNA in biliary epithelial cells is associated with the pathogenesis of biliary atresia. *Hepatology* 46(4): 1146-1154. (2007).

Hausherr-Bohn, Amparo: *Cellular and molecular characterization of novel lipopeptides with anti-myeloma activities*, Dissertation, Ludwig-Maximilians-Universität, München, 2009.

Hengartner MO. The biochemistry of apoptosis. *Nature* 407: 770-776. (2000).

Hopkins-Donaldson S, Bodmer JL, Bourloud KB, Brognara CB, Tschopp J and Gross N. Loss of caspase-8 expression in highly malignant human neuroblastoma cells correlates with resistance to tumor necrosis factor-related apoptosis-inducing ligand-induced apoptosis. *Cancer Res* 60(16): 4315-4319. (2000).

Hosaka S, Nakatsura T, Tsukamoto H, Hatayama T, Baba H, Nishimura Y. Synthetic small interfering RNA targeting heat shock protein 105 induces apoptosis of various cancer cells both in vitro and in vivo. *Cancer Sci* 97(7):623-32. (2006).

Ishikawa E, Nakazawa M, Yoshinari M and Minami M. Role of tumor necrosis factor-related apoptosis-inducing ligand in immune response to influenza virus infection in mice. *J Virol* 79(12): 7658-7663. (2005).

Ishimura N, Isomoto H, Bronk SF and Gores GJ. Trail induces cell migration and invasion in apoptosis-resistant cholangiocarcinoma cells. *Am J Physiol Gastrointest Liver Physiol* 290(1): 129-136. (2006).

Jackson AL, Burchard J, Schelter J, Chau BN, Cleary M, Lim L and Linsley PS. Position-specific chemical modification of siRNAs reduces "off-target" transcript silencing. *RNA* 12(7): 1179-1187. (2006).

Jeremias I and Debatin KM. TRAIL induces apoptosis and activation of NF-kappaB. *Eur Cytokine Netw* 9(4): 687-688. (1998).

References

Jo M, Kim TH, Seol DW, Esplen JE, Dorko K, Billiar TR and Strom SC. Apoptosis induced in normal human hepatocytes by tumor necrosis factor-related apoptosis-inducing ligand. *Nat Med* 6(5): 564-567. (2000).

Kallansrud G and Ward B. A comparison of measured and calculated single- and double- stranded oligodeoxynucleotide extinction coefficients. *Anal Biochem* 236(1): 134-138. (1996).

Karin M, Cao Y, Greten FR and Li ZW. NF-kappaB in cancer: from innocent bystander to major culprit. *Nat Rev Cancer* 2(4):301-310. (2002).

Kayagaki N, Yamaguchi N, Nakayama M, Kawasaki A, Akiba H, Okumura K and Yagita H. Involvement of TNF-related apoptosis-inducing ligand in human CD4+ T cell-mediated cytotoxicity. *J Immunol* 162(5): 2639-2647. (1999).

Kayagaki N, Yamaguchi N, Nakayama M, Takeda K, Akiba H, Tsutsui H, Okamura H, Nakanishi K, Okumura K and Yagita H. Expression and function of TNF-related apoptosis-inducing ligand on murine activated NK cells. *J Immunol*, 163(4): 1906-1913. (1999).

Keane MM, Ettenberg SA, Nau MM, Russell EK and Lipkowitz S. Chemotherapy augments TRAIL-induced apoptosis in breast cell lines. *Cancer Res* 59(3): 734-741. (1999).

Kelley SK, Harris LA, Xie D, DeForge L, Totpal K, Bussiere J and Fox JA. Preclinical studies to predict the disposition of Apo2L/tumor necrosis factor-related apoptosis-inducing ligand in humans: characterization of in vivo efficacy, pharmacokinetics, and safety. *J Pharmacol Exp Ther* 299(1): 31-38. (2001).

Kim K, Fisher MJ, Xu SQ and el-Deiry WS. Molecular determinants of response to TRAIL in killing of normal and cancer cells. *Clin Cancer Res* 6(2): 335-346. (2000).

Kimberley FC and Screaton GR. Following a TRAIL: update on a ligand and its five receptors. *Cell Res* 14(5): 359-372. (2004).

Kirstein M, Baglioni C. Tumor necrosis factor stimulates proliferation of human osteosarcoma cells and accumulation of c-myc messenger RNA. *J Cell Physiol* 134(3):479-84. (1988).

Kischkel FC, Hellbardt S, Behrmann I, Germer M, Pawlita M, Krammer PH and Peter ME. Cytotoxicity-dependent APO-1 (Fas/CD95)-associated proteins form a death-inducing signaling complex (DISC) with its receptor. *EMBO J* 14(22): 5579-5588. (1995).

Kroll, Lisa: Etablierung und Optimierung von Methoden zur Untersuchung der Wirkung von endogenem TRAIL als Wachstumsfaktor in Tumorzellen. *Dissertation.* Ludwig-Maximilians-Universität, München. 2012.

Lamhamedi-Cherradi SE, Zheng SJ, Maguschak KA, Peschon J and Chen YH. Defective thymocyte apoptosis and accelerated autoimmune disease in TRAIL -/- mice. *Nat Immunol* 4: 255-260. (2003).

Lancaster JM, Sayer R, Blanchette C, Calingaert B, Whitaker R, Schildkraut J, Marks J and Berchuck A. High expression of tumor necrosis factor-related apoptosis-inducing ligand is associated with favorable ovarian cancer survival. *Clin Cancer Res* 9(2): 762-766. (2003).

LeBlanc HN and Ashkenazi A. Apo2L/TRAIL and its death and decoy receptors. *Cell Death Differ* 10(1): 66-75. (2003).

References

Levina V, Marrangoni AM, DeMarco R, Gorelik E and Lokshin AE. Multiple effects of TRAIL in human carcinoma cells: induction of apoptosis, senescence, proliferation, and cytokine production. *Exp Cell Res* 314(7): 1605-1616. (2008).

Lin Y, Devin A, Cook A, Keane MM, Kelliher M, Lipkowitz S and Liu ZG. The death domain kinase RIP is essential for TRAIL (Apo2L)-induced activation of IkappaB kinase and c-Jun N-terminal kinase. *Mol Cell Biol* 20(18): 6638-6645. (2000).

Macher-Goeppinger S, Aulmann S, Tagscherer KE, Wagener N, Haferkamp A, Penzel R, Brauckhoff A, Hohenfellner M, Sykora J, Walczak H, Teh BT, Autschbach F, Herpel E, Schirmacher P and Roth W. Prognostic value of tumor necrosis factor-related apoptosis-inducing ligand (TRAIL) and TRAIL receptors in renal cell cancer. *Clin Cancer Res* 15(2): 650-659. (2009).

Maduro JH, Noordhuis MG, Ten Hoor KA, Pras E, Arts HJ, Eijsink JJ, Hollema H, Mom CH, de JS, de Vries EG, de Bock GH and van der Zee AG. The prognostic value of TRAIL and its death receptors in cervical cancer. *Int J Radiat Oncol Biol Phys* 75(1): 203-211. (2009).

Malhi H and Gores GJ. TRAIL resistance results in cancer progression: a TRAIL to perdition? *Oncogene* 25(56): 7333-7335. (2006).

Marsters SA, Sheridan JP, Pitti RM, Huang A, Skubatch M, Baldwin D, Yuan J, Gurney A, Goddard AD, Godowski P and Ashkenazi A. A novel receptor for ApoL/TRAIL contains a truncated death domain. *Curr Biol* 7(12): 1003-1006. (1997).

Martin-Villalba A, Herr I, Jeremias I, Hahne M, Brandt R, Vogel J, Schenkel J, Herdegen T and Debatin KM. CD95 ligand (Fas-L/APO-1L) and tumor necrosis factor-related apoptosis-inducing ligand mediate ischemia-induced apoptosis in neurons. *J Neurosci* 19(10): 3809-3817. (1999).

Martinez-Lorenzo MJ, Anel A, Gamen S, Monle n I, Lasierra P, Larrad L, Pineiro A, Alava MA and Naval J. Activated human T cells release bioactive Fas ligand and APO2 ligand in microvesicles. *J Immunol* 163(3): 1274-1281. (1999).

Mitsiades CS, Treon SP, Mitsiades N, Shima Y, Richardson P, Schlossman R, Hideshima T and Anderson KC. TRAIL/Apo2L ligand selectively induces apoptosis and overcomes drug resistance in multiple myeloma: therapeutic applications. *Blood* 98(3): 795-804. (2001).

Mongkolsapaya J, Grimes JM, Chen N, Xu XN, Stuart DI, Jones EY and Screaton GR. Structure of the TRAIL-DR5 complex reveals mechanisms conferring specificity in apoptotic initiation. *Nat Struct Biol* 6(11): 1048-1053. (1999).

Morel J, Audo R, Hahne M and Combe B. Tumor necrosis factor-related apoptosis-inducing ligand (TRAIL) induces rheumatoid arthritis synovial fibroblst proliferation through mitogen-activated protein kinases and phosphatidylinositol 3-kinase/Akt. *J Biol Chem* 280(16): 15709-15718. (2005).

Nagane M, Pan G, Weddle JJ, Dixit VM, Cavenee WK and Huang HJ. Increased death receptor 5 expression by chemotherapeutic agent in human gliomas cases synergistic cytotoxicity with tumor necrosis factor-related apoptosis-inducing ligand in vitro and in vivo. *Cancer Res* 60(4): 847-853. (2000).

Neubauer A, Wolf M, Engenhart-Cabillic R and Rothmund M. [Function and responsibility of an interdisciplinary tumor center. Need for a "cancer center" for multimodal therapy concepts]. *Dtsch Med Wochenschr* 127(17): 901-906. (2002).

References

Nicoletti I, Migliorati G, Pagliacci MC, Grignani F and Riccardi C. A rapid and simple method for measuring thymocyte apoptosis by propidium iodide staining and flow cytometry. *J Immunol Methods* 139(2): 271-279. (1991).

Ovcharenko D, Jarvis R, Hunicke-Smith S, Kelnar K and Brown D. High-throughput RNAi screening in vitro: from cell lines to primary cells. *RNA* 11(6): 985-993. (2005).

Oya M, Ohtsubo M, Takayanagi A, Tachibana M, Shimizu N, Murai M. Constitutive activation of nuclear factor-kappaB prevents TRAIL-induced apoptosis in renal cancer cells. *Oncogene* 20(29):3888-96. (2001).

Pan G, O'Rourke K, Chinnaiyan AM, Gentz R, Ebner R, Ni J and Dixit VM. The receptor for the cytotoxic ligand TRAIL. *Science* 276(5309): 111-113. (1997).

Papac RJ. Origins of cancer therapy. *Yale J Biol Med* 74(6): 391-398. (2001).

Pfaffl MW. A new mathematical model for relative quantification in real-time RT-PCR. *Nucleic Acids Res* 29(9): e45. (2001).

Pitti RM, Marsters SA, Ruppert S, Donahue CJ, Moore A and Ashkenazi A. Induction of apoptosis by Apo-2 ligand, a new member of the tumour necrosis factor cytokine family. *J Biol Chem* 271(22): 12687-12690. (1996).

Robertson NM, Zangrilli JG, Steplewski A, Hastie A, Lindemeyer RG, Planeta MA, Smith MK, Innocent N, Musani A, Pascual R, Peters S and Litwack G. Differential expression of TRAIL and TRAIL receptors in allergic asthmatics following segmental antigen challenge: evidence for a role of TRAIL in eosinophil survival. *J Immunol,* 169(10): 5986-5996. (2002).

Rogers PR, Song J, Gramaglia I, Killeen N, Croft M. OX40 promotes Bcl-xL and Bcl-2 expression and is essential for long-term survival of CD4 T cells. *Immunity* 15:445–455. (2001).

Ross RA and Spengler BA. The conundrum posed by cellular heterogeneity in analysis of human neuroblastoma. *J Natl Cancer Inst* 96(16): 1192-1193. (2004).

Roth W, Isenmann S, Naumann U, Kugler S, Bahr M, Dichgans J, Ashkenazi A and Weller M. Locoregional Apo2L/TRAIL eradicates intracranial human malignant glioma xenografts in athymic mice in the absence of neurotoxicity. *Biochem Biophys Res Commun* 265(2): 479-483. (1999).

Saelens X, Festjens N, Vande WL, van GM, van LG and Vandenabeele P. Toxic proteins released from mitochondria in cell death. *Oncogene* 23(16): 2861-2874. (2004).

Sanlioglu AD, Dirice E, Elpek O, Korcum AF, Balci MK, Omer A, Griffith TS and Sanlioglu S. High levels of endogenous tumor necrosis factor-related apoptosis-inducing ligand expression correlate with increased cell death in human pancreas. *Pancreas* 36(4): 385-393. (2008).

Secchiero P, Gonelli A, Carnevale E, Corallini F, Rizzardi C, Zacchigna S, Melato M and Zauli G. Evidence for a proangiogenic activity of TNF-related apoptosis-inducing ligand. *Neoplasia* 6(4): 364-373. (2004).

Secchiero P, Gonelli A, Carnevale E, Milani D, Pandolfi A, Zella D and Zauli G. TRAIL promotes the survival and proliferation of primary human vascular endothelial cells by activating the Akt and ERK pathways. *Circulation,* 107(17): 2250-2256. (2003).

References

Sedger LM, Glaccum MB, Schuh JC, Kanaly ST, Williamson E, Kayagaki N, Yun T, Smolak P, Le T, Goodwin R and Gliniak B. Characterization of the in vivo function of TNF-alpha-related apoptosis-inducing ligand, TRAIL/Apo2L, using TRAIL/Apo2L gene-deficient mice. *Eur J Immunol* 32(8): 2246-2254. (2002).

Sheridan JP, Marsters SA, Pitti RM, Gurney A, Skubatch M, Baldwin D, Ramakrishnan L, Gray CL, Baker K, Wood WI, Goddard AD, Godowski P and Ashkenazi A. Control of TRAIL-induced apoptosis by a family of signaling and decoy receptors. *Science* 277(5327): 818-821. (1997).

Shetty S, Gladden JB, Henson ES, Hu X, Villanueva J, Haney N and Gibson SB. Tumor necrosis factor-related apoptosis inducing ligand (TRAIL) up-regulates death receptor 5 (DR5) mediated by NFkappaB activation in epithelial derived cell lines. *Apoptosis* 7(5): 413-420. (2002).

Shi J, Zheng D, Liu Y, Sham MH, Tam P, Farzaneh F and Xu R. Overexpression of soluble TRAIL induces apoptosis in human lung adenocarcinoma and inhibits growth of tumor xenografts in nude mice. *Cancer Res* 65(5): 1687-1692. (2005).

Smyth MJ, Cretney E, Takeda K, Wiltrout RH, Sedger LM, Kayagaki N, Yagita H and Okumura K. Tumor necrosis factor-related apoptosis-inducing ligand (TRAIL) contributes to interferon gamma-dependent natural killer cell protection from tumor metastasis. *J Exp Med* 193(6): 661-670. (2001).

Spierings DC, de Vries EG, Timens W, Groen HJ, Boezen HM and de JS. Expression of TRAIL and TRAIL death receptors in stage III non-small cell lung cancer tumors. *Clin Cancer Res* 9(9): 3397-3405. (2003).

Spierings DC, de Vries EG, Vellenga E, van den Heuvel FA, Koornstra JJ, Wesseling J, Hollema H and de JS. Tissue distribution of the death ligand TRAIL and its receptors. *J Histochem Cytochem* 52(6): 821-831. (2004).

Sprick MR, Weigand MA, Rieser E, Rauch CT, Juo P, Blenis J, Krammer PH and Walczak H. FADD/MORT1 and caspase-8 are recruited to TRAIL receptors 1 and 2 are essential for apoptosis mediated by TRAIL receptor 2. *Immunity* 12(6): 599-609. (2000).

Street SE, Cretney E and Smyth MJ. Perforin and interferon-gamma activities independently control tumor initiation, growth and metastasis. *Blood* 97(1): 192-197. (2001).

Takeda K, Smyth MJ, Cretney E, Hayakawa Y, Kayagaki N, Yagita H and Okumura K. Critical role for tumor necrosis factor-related apoptosis-inducing ligand in immune surveillance against tumor development. *J Exp Med* 195(2): 161-169. (2002).

Tong AW, Zhang YA, Nemunaitis J. Small interfering RNA for experimental cancer therapy. *Curr Opin Mol Ther* 7(2):114-24. (2005).

Trauzold A, Siegmund D, Schniewind B, Sipos B, Egberts J, Zorenkov D, Emme D, Roder C, Kalthoff H and Wajant H. *Oncogene:* 25: 7434-7439. (2006).

Tselepis C, Perry I, Dawson C, Hardy R, Darnton SJ, McConkey C, Stuart RC, Wright N, Harrison R, Jankowski JA. Tumour necrosis factor-alpha in Barrett's oesophagus: a potential novel mechanism of action. *Oncogene* 21(39):6071-81. (2002).

Ui-Tei K, Naito Y and Saigo K. Guidelines for the selection of effective short-interfering RNA sequences for functional genomics. *Methods Mol Biol* 361: 201-216. (2007).

References

Van Geelen CM, Westra JL, de Vries EG, Boersma-van EW, Zwart N, Hollema H, Boezen HM, Mulder NH, Plukker JT, de JS, Kleibeuker JH and Koornstra JJ. Prognostic significance of tumor necrosis factor-related apoptosis-inducing ligand and its receptors in adjuvantly treated stage III colon cancer patients. *J Clin Oncol* 24: 4998-5004. (2006).

Van Poznak C, Cross SS, Saggese M, Hudis C, Panageas KS, Norton L, Coleman RE and Holen I. Expression of osteoprotergin (OPG), TNF related apoptosis inducing ligand (TRAIL), and receptors activator of nuclear factor kappaB ligand (RANKL) in human breast tumours. *J Clin Pathol* 59: 56-63. (2006).

Vilimanovich U, Bumbasirevic V. TRAIL induces proliferation of human glioma cells by c-FLIPL-mediated activation of ERK1/2. *Cell Mol Life Sci* 65(5):814-26. (2008).

Vinay DS, Kwon BS. TNF superfamily: costimulation and clinical applications. *Cell Biol Int* 33(4):453-65. (2009).

Walczak H, Miller RE, Ariail K, Gliniak B, Griffith TS, Kubin M, Chin W, Jones J, Woodward A, Le T, Smith C, Smolak P, Goodwin RG, Rauch CT, Schuh JC and Lynch DH. Tumoricidal activity of tumor necrosis factor-related apoptosis-inducing ligand in vivo. *Nat Med* 5(2): 157-163. (1999).

Walczak H, Krammer PH. The CD95 (APO-1/Fas) and the TRAIL (APO-2L) apoptosis systems. *Exp Cell Res* 256(1):58-66. (2000).

Weckmann M, Collison A, Simpson JL, Kopp MV, Wark PA, Smyth MJ, Yagita H, Matthaei KI, Hansbro N, Whitehead B, Gibson PG, Foster PS and Mattes J. Critical link between TRAIL and CCL20 for the activation of TH2 cells and the expression of allergic airway disease. *Nat Med* 13(11): 1308-1315. (2007).

Wen J, Ramadevi N, Nguyen D, Perkins C, Worthington E and Bhalla K. Antileukemic drugs increase ddeath receptor 5 levels and enhance Apo-2L-induced apoptosis of human acute leukemia cells. *Blood* 96(12): 3900-3906. (2000).

Wiley SR, Schooley K, Smolak PJ, Din WS, Huang CP, Nicholl JK, Sutherland GR, Smith TD, Rauch C, Smith CA et al. Identification and characterization of a new member of the TNF family that induces apoptosis. *Immunity* 3(6): 673-682. (1995).

Wu W, Hodges E, Redelius J and Hoog C. A novel approach for evaluating the efficiency of siRNAs on protein levels in cultured cells. *Nucleic Acids Res* 32(2): e17. (2004).

Wyllie AH, Kerr JF and Currie AR. Cell death: the significance of apoptosis. *Int Rev Cytol* 68: 251-306. (1980).

Yoshida T, Zhang Y, Rivera Rosado LA and Zhang B. Repeated treatment with subtoxic doses of TRAIL induces resistance to apoptosis through its death receptors in MDA-MB-231 breast cancer cells. *Mol Cancer Res* 7(11): 1835-1844. (2009).

Zauli G, Sancilio S, Cataldi A, Sabatini N, Bosco D and Di PR. PI-3K/Akt and NF-kappaB/IkappaBalpha pathways are activated in Jurkat T cells in response to TRAIL treatment. *J Cell Physiol* 202(3): 900-911. (2005).

Zhang XD, Franco AV, Nguyen T, Gray CP, Hersey P. Differential localization and regulation of death and decoy receptors for TNF-related apoptosis-inducing ligand (TRAIL) in human melanoma cells. *J Immunology* 164(8): 3961-70. (2000).

11 Acknowledgement

I would like to thank my direct supervisor, PD. Dr. med. Irmela Jeremias, for giving me an interesting topic to work on and the possibility to work in a motivating scientific environment. Thank you for opening the world of research to me.

I want to thank Dr. med. Harald Ehrhardt and Dr. Nadja Tediskaya for the interesting thematic discussions.

I want to thank Lisa Kroll for laying the methodical foundation for the present work. Many thanks to Michaela Grunert, Ines Höfig and Sibylle Gündisch for their professional support in everyday bench work. Your friendship and professional collaboration was very important to me.

Special thanks to Naschla Kohistani for her friendship, inspiring discussions and friendly support during harder times.

For the many hours supporting and encouraging me to finish this work I want to thank Viktor Kölzer. You inspire me.

12 Publication

Parts of the present work were published as abstract and presented at the following symposium:

Brittingham S, Kroll L, Jeremias I. *Role of endogenous TRAIL for tumor cell growth.* "Advances in Cell Death Research", Apoptrain Symposium, Günzburg, Germany, 2008, Poster, Abstract° 22, Page

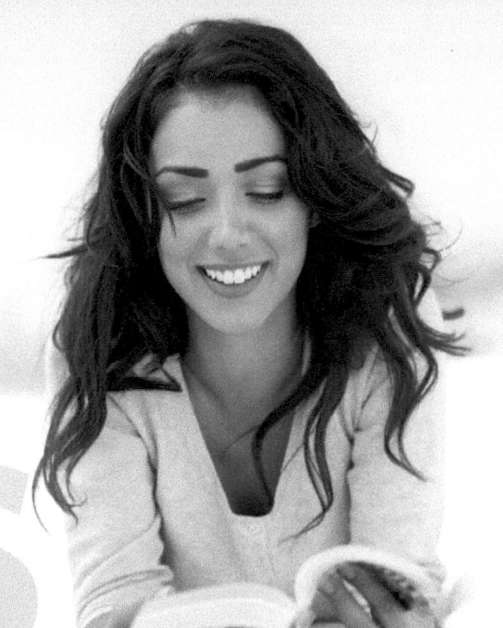

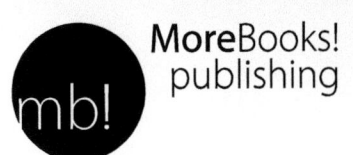

i want morebooks!

Buy your books fast and straightforward online - at one of world's fastest growing online book stores! Environmentally sound due to Print-on-Demand technologies.

Buy your books online at
www.get-morebooks.com

Kaufen Sie Ihre Bücher schnell und unkompliziert online – auf einer der am schnellsten wachsenden Buchhandelsplattformen weltweit! Dank Print-On-Demand umwelt- und ressourcenschonend produziert.

Bücher schneller online kaufen
www.morebooks.de

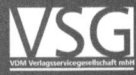

VDM Verlagsservicegesellschaft mbH
Heinrich-Böcking-Str. 6-8   Telefon: +49 681 3720 174   info@vdm-vsg.de
D - 66121 Saarbrücken   Telefax: +49 681 3720 1749   www.vdm-vsg.de

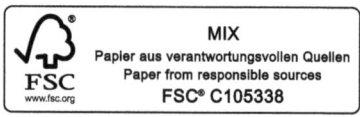

Printed by Books on Demand GmbH, Norderstedt / Germany